616.1
DEF

DeFelice,
Stephen L., 1936-
    The carnitine
defense

DEC 21 1999

DATE			

"Dr. DeFelice's findings are wide-ranging. I applaud his continuing fascination with carnitine's potential role in health maintenance and, more broadly, the evidence favoring the benefits of such other nutraceuticals as folate and vitamin E."

Peter Goldman, M.D., Professor of Health Science
Department of Nutrition, Harvard Medical School

"Dr. DeFelice is the father of the term 'nutraceutical.' The primary, but not exclusive, purpose of nutraceuticals such as carnitine is to prevent disease whereas the overwhelming aim of medicine is to treat it."

Paul A. Lachance, Ph.D., D.Sc., Executive Director
The Nutraceuticals Institute of Rutgers University
and St. Joseph's University

"Dr. DeFelice has pulled together an amazing amount of controversial data on the relation of nutrition to cardiovascular disease. Many readers will end up better informed about these important matters."

Louis Lasagna, M.D., Dean
Sackler School of Graduate Biomedical Sciences
Tufts University

"Written in a thoughtful yet straightforward manner, Dr. DeFelice sets things into perspective. He is a thought leader in this field, going beyond the well-worn, politically correct solutions that haven't worked as we expected."

Lawrence M. Resnick, M.D.
Professor of Medicine, Director of Hypertension
Wayne State University Medical Center, Detroit, MI

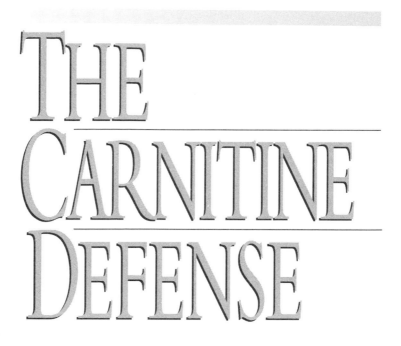

THE
CARNITINE
DEFENSE

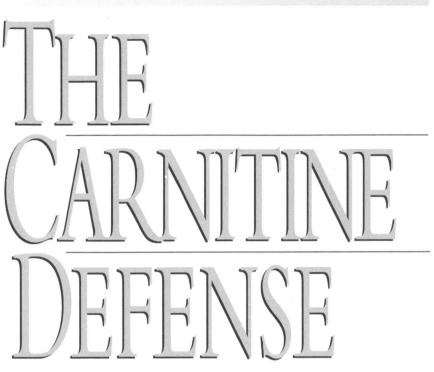

THE CARNITINE DEFENSE

A **Nutraceutical** Formula
to Prevent and Treat
Heart Disease, the Nation's #1 Killer

Stephen L. DeFelice, M.D.
with Helen Kohl

RODALE

REACH™

Printed in the United States of America on acid-free ∞ , recycled paper ♻

Cover and Interior Designer: Christopher Rhoads
Interior Illustrator: Molly Babich

Library of Congress Cataloging-in-Publication Data

DeFelice, Stephen L., 1936–
 The carnitine defense : a nutraceutical formula to prevent and treat heart disease, the nation's #1 killer / Stephen L. DeFelice, with Helen Kohl.
  p. ; cm.
 Includes index.
 ISBN 1–57954–133–X hardcover
 1. Carnitine—Therapeutic use. 2. Coronary heart disease—Prevention. 3. Coronary heart disease—Alternative treatment. 4. Functional foods. I. Kohl, Helen. II. Title.
 [DNLM: 1. Carnitine—therapeutic use. 2. Dietary Supplements. 3. Heart Diseases—prevention & control. 4. Heart Diseases—therapy. QU 187 D313c 1999]
 RC685.C6 D4235 1999
 616.1'061—dc21   99–046985

Distributed to the book trade by St. Martin's Press

2 4 6 8 10 9 7 5 3 1 hardcover

Visit us on the Web at www.rodalebooks.com, or call us toll-free at (800) 848-4735.

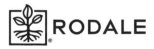

RODALE

WE INSPIRE AND ENABLE PEOPLE TO IMPROVE
THEIR LIVES AND THE WORLD AROUND THEM

Notice

This book is intended as a reference volume only, not as a medical manual. The information given here is designed to help you make informed decisions about your health. It is not intended as a substitute for any treatment that may have been prescribed by your doctor. If you suspect that you have a medical problem, we urge you to seek competent medical help.

This book is dedicated to the memory of James Vick, Ph.D. Shortly after the final chapter of this book was written, my good friend and colleague, Colonel James Vick, was killed in a tragic accident.

Colonel Vick, when he was the young and dynamic Major Vick, played a crucial role in helping me with the critical early phases of carnitine research.

This book is dedicated to the memory of this kind man.

Acknowledgments

Many people encouraged and helped me in bringing about the Nutraceutical Revolution and in writing this book. Two men in particular, Louis Lasagna, M.D., and Stephen H. McNamara, Esq., stood by my side in the very difficult beginning, in my efforts to launch this very critical nutraceutical message: It is important to demonstrate in clinical studies that foods and dietary supplements that people consume have beneficial health effects such as the prevention and/or treatment of disease.

A particular note of gratitude for my research colleagues in the food industry go to Alfred S. Cummin, Ph.D.; Enrique J. Guardia, Ph.D.; and Robert E. Smith, Ph.D.; who, with little support from their colleagues, encouraged me to move forward with the Nutraceutical Revolution.

To others who also lent a helping hand and to those who spent the time to critique the text of this book, I wish to thank Nilo Cater, M.D.; Lyn Ciocca; Susan Clarey; Doug Dollemore; Joseph R. DiPalma, M.D.; Kathy Everleth; Claire Gerus; Peter Goldman, M.D.; Paul A. Lachance, Ph.D.; Louis Lasagna, M.D.; Michael Mannion; Jerry Nadler, M.D.; Hugh O'Neill; Lawrence M. Resnick, M.D.; Eric B. Rimm, Sc.D.; Richard S. Rivlin, M.D.; George F. Schreiner, M.D., Ph.D.; Jay S. Skyler, M.D; and Meir Stampfer, M.D.

A special thanks to Antonio C. Martinez II, Esq., for helping me educate our colleagues in Washington, D.C., regarding the importance of nutraceutical research, and to Senator Bill Frist, M.D. (R–TN), Senator Tom Harkin (D–IA), Representative Frank Pallone (D–NJ), and Patricia Knight, Chief of Staff to Senator Orrin Hatch (R–UT), for their support in achieving this goal.

There are two gentlemen who deserve very special consideration: Claudio Cavazza, Ph.D., and James Vick, Ph.D. Dr. Vick, as a Major in the U.S. Army at the Walter Reed Army Institute of Research in Washington, D.C., was largely responsible for performing early animal experiments to demonstrate carnitine's potential medical benefits. Dr. Cavazza, the proprietor of the pharmaceutical company Sigma Tau, based in Pomezia, Italy, is the man who took the chance and sponsored most of the important clinical studies on carnitine.

Additional special thanks to Elizabeth Meehan and Patricia Park is more than deserved for keeping my wandering mind from going astray. It's not easy, I can assure you.

This book would not have been possible without the laborious effort of my co-author, Helen Kohl. Her admirable tenacity in revising draft after draft saved me from despair.

And finally, in the past, I promised my wife, Patrice, that I would never write a book again. What she didn't know is that one hand was behind my back when I said it—with my fingers crossed!

—Stephen L. DeFelice, M.D.

I got my first tantalizing glimpse into the tremendous health potential for nutraceuticals at Dr. DeFelice's Foundation for Innovation in Medicine conference held in Washington, D.C., in November 1997. I was deeply impressed with Dr. DeFelice's knowledge, his dedication in accumulating such a compelling body of evidence, and the expertise of his speakers. Little did I know that that glimpse was the beginning of a veritable roller-coaster ride through cutting-edge health research around the world. I'd like to thank Dr. DeFelice for the trip, as well as his dedicated and hardworking assistants, Elizabeth Meehan and Patricia Park. Rodale's hardworking staff—Sally Reith and Lois Hazel, in particular—scoured the Internet and the nation's research libraries for the latest and best information; Alisa Bauman and Hugh O'Neill provided valuable editorial input; and my editor, Susan Clarey, kept me strong, made me laugh, and infused this book with her words of wisdom. My agent, Claire Gerus, put this deal together; she also held me together. And my husband, Christopher Clayton, along with our children, Ryan and Laurel Clayton, not only kept the home fires aglow but also provided what every writer needs: honest feedback laced with unconditional support.

—Helen Kohl

Foreword

The public's interest in the relationship of nutrition to good health seems to grow with each passing day. People want answers to many questions but are often confused by mixed messages from the media and from the scientific literature. Is the American diet (whatever that may be!) good enough? Do I need to take dietary supplements? Is the generally recommended daily intake of nutrients on target, or too low? Can I harm myself by taking nutritional supplements? Who can I believe?

Medical school training has traditionally pooh-poohed concerns that our national diet is suboptimal, despite abundant evidence that food intake is for many of our citizens capricious or even bizarre.

Stephen L. DeFelice, M.D., a physician who is a pharmaceutical as well as a nutraceutical expert, has for years been trying to cut a path through the nutritional wilderness. He coined the word *nutraceutical*. He regularly convenes well-attended meetings to debate these issues. In this book, he has pulled together a lot of information (often contradictory) and given the reader his working philosophy. The available data, as Dr. DeFelice points out, defy simplistic analysis. The reader may not agree with Dr. DeFelice's conclusions, but his argument deserves careful scrutiny. More and more physicians, however, are joining the DeFelice bandwagon.

Important for both physicians and patients, there is no possibility of agnosticism here. If one chooses not to take nutritional supplements, one is not withholding judgment, but rather betting that the supplements will not prove helpful. The opposite is true for "believers"—they are betting that the supplements are likely to help. It is like Pascal's wager re the existence of God. If one bets against God and he really exists, the penalty is a frightening fate. Whereas, if God does not exist and one mistakenly believes that he does, so what? I wonder what Pascal's heavenly ghost would advise us today about *The Carnitine Defense*.

Louis Lasagna, M.D.
Dean, Sackler School of Graduate Biomedical Sciences
Tufts University

Contents

Part One: The Case for Carnitine

Part Two: The Cardiac Elixir

Part Three: Beyond Carnitine

Why I Wrote This Book

We all know it, and let's face it: The pace and environment of modern society are playing increasingly major roles as causes of heart disease. Stress and foreign substances that we breathe and consume are everywhere. Emotional stress is almost constant. Women are working and tired—especially those with children. Men can expect to have four or five jobs during their career paths, hardly a foundation for security and peace of mind. Couple all of this with the now common and traumatic stress of divorce, and it is self-evident that emotional stress is now a way of life, negatively impacting our cardiovascular systems as well as other factors that contribute to a good quality of life. Cardiac tranquillity may exist on Crete where there is very little cardiac disease, but not in our great country.

How are we eating? Obesity in the United States is rampant. People are grabbing meals on the run, frequently consuming unhealthy, unbalanced meals, as well as completely missing the beauty and tranquillity that accompany a good meal, good wine, and good company. And many of us are now paying the price of increasing mobility and these abysmal eating habits. Heart disease marches on as the number one killer in the United States. In the past, this book would have been directed toward men. Heart disease was almost solely in the domain of men. Now, it is very rapidly on its way to being as common and as devastating in women.

There is, however, some very good news. We have now entered an exciting new era of medicine—nutraceuticals. "Nutraceuticals" essentially include foods and dietary supplements. You can get vitamin C in a fresh orange or in a pill—both are nutraceuticals. The good news is that cardiovascular nutraceuticals, both to prevent and treat heart disease, are showing breathtaking promise.

We all know, at least we aging folk, that when there is promise, there are problems. Many Americans are taking the cardiovascular nutraceuticals without proper guidance from their physicians. As a result, many may not be obtaining the optimum benefits offered by cardiovascular nutraceuticals. There is, therefore, an urgent need for this book as a guide to both you and your physicians on what, why, and how much to take.

The conclusion of the book is that cardiovascular nutraceuticals should generally be taken in combinations and not as single substances. I call the specific combination in this book the Cardiac Elixir. Many factors cause cardiovascular disease leading to heart attacks. It makes good sense, therefore, to combat these factors with a mixture of nutraceuticals that attacks these processes.

Carnitine is the centerpiece of the Cardiac Elixir. It acts in your heart to protect it against a lack of oxygen, or myocardial ischemia. There are numerous well-done clinical studies that demonstrate this effect. Carnitine probably will be news to you, but it is good news.

The recommendations in this book are based primarily on published clinical studies and the opinions of medical experts. After all, it makes good sense to test nutraceuticals in people to determine whether they work rather than to recommend them based on animal studies alone. Nutraceuticals tested in animals should be given to animals and not to people. The more good clinical data available, the stronger a recommendation I will give.

I can assure you that new studies on the heart benefits of nutraceuticals will be published at a rapid pace within the near future. These studies will definitely affect the recommended ingredients in the second-generation Cardiac Elixir.

In this book, I frequently advise you to communicate with your physician about taking cardiovascular nutraceuticals, whether they are mentioned in this book or not, particularly if you are taking pharmaceuticals or drugs for your heart disease. The time has come for a nutraceutical partnership between the patient and the doctor, whether dealing with prevention or treatment. We are all patients—or potential ones, trying to ward off the fatal thud of a heart attack. This is the goal of mainstream medicine. I strongly advise you to join it.

—Stephen L. DeFelice, M.D.

PART ONE

The Case for Carnitine

CHAPTER ONE

Carnitine, Nature, and Defending Our Hearts

Carnitine. You've probably never heard the word. But carnitine, a natural proteinlike substance manufactured by our livers and kidneys out of two amino acids, is the world's best-kept nutraceutical secret. I believe that carnitine can offer protection for our hearts and that many of us should take carnitine supplements daily.

Carnitine's job is to carry fatty acids, a powerful source of fuel, into our mitochondria, the structures in our cells that produce energy. Carnitine has been called a steam-shovel molecule because it fills these cellular furnaces and lets us turn fuel into the energy that we need to breathe, walk around, play golf, rake the lawn, and even lie on the couch and watch television.

Carnitine, taken in supplement form, can not only help prevent damage that leads to heart disease but also provide lifesaving benefits for people who already have cardiovascular problems as well as protection for millions of perfectly healthy people who are, without knowing it, at risk of heart attack. Further, there is strong evidence that carnitine is just one in a group of natural substances that, when taken together in supplement form, can offer protection against the onset or progression of heart disease. This combination of substances forms the Cardiac Elixir at the heart of this book.

If you've read this far, you're probably already trying to live a life free from heart disease. You're probably trying to stick to a low-fat, low-cholesterol diet. You may be on cholesterol-lowering medication. You probably get some regular aerobic exercise. You may even manage your stress level through meditation or yoga or whatever helps you relax.

You're doing everything you can do to prevent heart disease, right? Wrong. There's more that you can do to protect yourself. There is compelling evidence reported in clinical studies and supported by medical experts that taking supplements of carnitine and other selected natural substances should become one of your health habits.

Mother Nature Is a Doctor's Best Friend

Mother Nature wants us to be well. Yes, she features plenty of dangers—from bacteria to typhoons—but she has also equipped us with remarkable defenses. An ingenious immune system, a thick skull to protect our brains, skin that heals itself, and bones that do, too. I have spent most of my career exploring and promoting the medicinal power of nature, specifically, how substances in our bodies and in foods can be used to prevent and treat disease.

My interest in nature's medicines dates from an unforgettable night, back when I was a third-year medical student at Jefferson Medical College in Philadelphia. I was getting tired of just studying anatomy and neurophysiology. I was eager to work with patients— to be a real doctor. So, I went to work in an understaffed emergency room in a rough section of the city, where violence and trauma were commonplace. I was a little apprehensive since I was just a student, but the hospital administrator assured me that there would always be a physician on call in case there was a situation that I couldn't handle. My first night proved the wisdom in the proverbial warning to be careful about what you wish for because you might get it. I got just what I thought I wanted: a crash course in hands-on medicine.

At first, things were unusually quiet in the emergency room. So, at 1:00 A.M., I decided to catch a nap. Back then, I was just a beginner and didn't know the rule that the surest way to bring in some emergency-room business was for the doctor to lie down and try to sleep. I had no sooner closed my eyes than I got an urgent call from the nurse.

"Hurry, doctor," she said. "We have a patient in critical condition."

I jumped up, splashed some water on my face, and rushed to the emergency room. As soon as the elevator doors opened, I heard the distinctive sound of a patient having a severe asthma attack. Though asthma attacks can still be quite serious, back then, they were an even more acute emergency. We gave this middle-aged man who was gasping for breath two hormones—adrenaline and steroids—along with the plant alkaloid theophylline at repeated intervals. Within a few hours, his condition was improved markedly.

Later that night, I made the mistake of trying to lie down again. "Doctor, hurry," the nurse said this time. "The police have delivered a comatose patient."

The man was in a diabetic coma. We gave him large doses of insulin, took some other therapeutic steps, and thereafter, he became conscious and recovered.

My third patient that night arrived to the wail of police sirens. A sobbing woman was carried in on a stretcher. She had her hands clasped over her face.

"What's the problem, officer?" I asked.

"Lye," he said. Somebody had thrown this highly corrosive substance in the woman's face.

The nurse quickly filled a basin with water, and we submerged the woman's head to dilute the lye. We repeated this periodically

Keeping the Clinical Research in Natural Medicine

These days, there's a lot of enthusiasm for so-called natural medicine. People are interested in ancient herbal remedies, food cures, and primitive healing arts that predate modern medicine. While I have no doubt that, in our techno-rush forward, we left behind some healing wisdom, I'm concerned that many proponents of natural medicine are driven by both an admiration of nature and a suspicion of technology and drugs.

I'd like to encourage the former and warn against the latter. While I bow to no man in my respect for nature's cures, we can't find them—and learn how to use them—without technology. There are good reasons to rummage through time-honored healing traditions for abandoned treasures. But it's vital that we resist merely nostalgic, unscientific thinking. Our enthusiasm for nature's medicines mustn't spring from a hostility to the science of medicine, as I fear it often does.

Do technology and nature sometimes conflict? Of course. The most obvious example is in how carelessly deployed technology has polluted the planet and may be responsible for epidemics of cancer and other diseases. In a way, the doctor-patient relationship has been diminished by technology as well. We could probably use fewer machines and more moments of care. But we mustn't let our disappointment with how modern medicine works—or, rather, doesn't work—make us content to dabble in unproven remedies, this herb-of-the-month, or that magic hormone that promises to fix everything that ails you.

Nature and modern medicine aren't enemies. In fact, one of the real goals of medicine is to figure out the technology of nature—how natural molecules work and how to access their health benefits. In my more philosophical moments, I think of medicine as the highest expression of one corner of nature: human nature.

for about an hour. Though I was pretty sure that the woman would have some facial scarring, I was also confident that the simple treatment with water would minimize it.

After my shift was over, I couldn't even think about sleeping. I was wired, enthused about the excitement of becoming a doctor. I went right to my classes the next morning without even sleeping. And it was only the next afternoon that the significant fact about my first night as a real doctor hit me: *All of those patients had been treated with natural substances.*

The adrenaline, steroids, and theophylline that had helped the asthma patient were natural medicines. The insulin that had treated the patient in diabetic coma was a natural medicine. And the water that had diluted the lye was a natural balm.

I was struck by the clash between the technological tone of the medical education I was getting and the fact that our most effective cures were natural. In the classroom, I was learning about powerful diagnostic machines and the scientific method and artificial drug molecules that could treat disease. But that night in the emergency room, nature had some impressive answers.

At the time, as a young man, the technology/nature split seemed like a conflict to me. Of course, within a few years, after I had finished school, I came to a more mature understanding. Technology and nature aren't really in opposition at all; technology is how we figure nature out. But that day, a seed was planted somewhere in my brain, a seed that remained dormant until I first encountered carnitine.

My First Glimpse of Carnitine's Healing Power

My history with carnitine goes back to my early days as a doctor. In 1961, after medical school, I studied at Jefferson Medical College as a National Institute of Health fellow in endocrinology (the study of glands, such as the pituitary and thyroid, which secrete hormones). Then I took a fellowship in clinical pharmacology at St. Vincent's Medical Center in New York City. Clinical pharmacology, translated into English, is the specialty that tests substances, be they natural or artificial, in humans to assess their medical value. In other words, do they help people or not?

Sheldon Gilgore, M.D., of Naples, Florida, former chairman of the pharmaceutical firm G.D. Searle and Company and former president of Pfizer, another pharmaceutical company, asked me to evaluate the clinical data for carnitine as a treatment for thyroid disease. At the time, I didn't know much about carnitine beyond the fact that it was a natural substance found in just about every cell in the body. But since I had been trained as an endocrinologist, thyroid disease was one of my areas of expertise. I agreed with Dr. Gilgore that the clinical studies on carnitine, though not well-done, were suggestive enough to warrant further investigation. I gave three women with classic symptoms of hyperthyroidism—excessive sweating, hand tremors, weight loss with nervousness, palpitations, increased appetite—supplemental carnitine. The results were surprisingly dramatic.

Within 2 weeks, the signs and symptoms of the disease virtually disappeared in all three women. Needless to say, I was tremendously excited. Here I was, just starting out, and the first small clinical study that I did had promising results. Not a bad first at-bat. But the results were less conclusive and more complex than they at first appeared. When we checked the hyperactivity of the patients' thyroid glands, we were surprised to find it unchanged from before they had been given the carnitine. That meant that if the carnitine had indeed somehow benefited them, it wasn't by acting on their thyroids. It had acted somewhere else in their bodies. But where? Exactly what had the supplemental carnitine done?

To this day, more than 35 years later, I can't say that I know exactly how to explain the results of that clinical study, though subsequent studies have shown that there is a definite thyroid hormone–carnitine connection. But whatever the explanation, that small study changed my life. I became intrigued by the medical promise of carnitine and launched a larger clinical trial. That study, conducted in a prison research unit, was designed to follow up on the findings of the first study, to see if carnitine could block excessive thyroid hormone activity. But, as often happens in medical research, I learned something entirely unexpected, or what you might call serendipity. This study offered my first hint that carnitine had potential as a heart or cardiac protector against ischemia, or reduced bloodflow to the heart. Shortly after he started taking carnitine supplements, one of the people in the study told me that for the first time in many years, he felt some relief from the chest pain of angina, the pain caused by lack of oxygen to the heart. Though nitroglycerin therapy and other standard treatments for angina in those days hadn't helped him much, he said that the carnitine significantly lessened his pain.

"Doc, it's a miracle," he said. "My chest pain is gone!"

That was my first inkling that carnitine could help the heart. I didn't know it then, but I was embarking upon a long, fascinating journey. Since my early seat-of-the-pants days, when I actually did experiments on myself and began to spread the word about natural medicines, I've initiated multiple clinical studies on the effect of carnitine on healthy people as well as on people with heart problems.

There is compelling scientific evidence that supplemental carnitine offers great cardiovascular benefits. It can not only help prevent heart disease but also help treat several heart problems, including myocardial ischemia, a lack of oxygen to the heart, and cardiomyopathy, a weak heart, in certain patients. Perhaps most important, there is strong clinical evidence to suggest that if you have a heart attack, high levels of carnitine in your system can minimize damage to your heart. I believe that for a significant number of people, taking carnitine supplements can be a lifesaving habit.

Carnitine is one of the best-kept nutraceutical secrets among nature's medicines. Neither physicians nor the public are aware of its enormous medicinal potential. In chapter 7, I explain carnitine's metabolic role in our bodies and its special importance to our hearts. I also explain how we medical researchers discovered that carnitine could be part of a cardiac insurance policy and exactly how to use it. But I want to emphasize that carnitine is just part of a larger health message. We can and must do more to protect our hearts. I believe that supplementation with natural substances is the next immediate great frontier of preventive cardiac care.

A New Weapon against Heart Disease

Nutraceutical.

Here's another word that you may never have heard. I coined and defined it because after a while, it became clear to me that we needed a single phrase to describe natural substances taken orally that keep us healthy. So I just combined the words *nutrient* and *pharmaceutical* and came up with *nutraceutical*, a new word for a broad class of natural substances that can keep us well or make us well. It caught on. The word *nutraceutical* has very long arms. It embraces foods and dietary supplements such as vitamins, minerals, hormones, and amino acids. An orange and pasta are examples of nutraceuticals; so are magnesium, garlic, and gingko biloba.

The Carnitine Defense is a combination of nutraceuticals, an elixir or mixture of natural molecules that will help prevent our greatest destructive illness: heart disease, the nation's number one killer. It's a cardiac health regimen whose time has come. Science has thrown lots of firepower at cardiovascular illness. The development of many different kinds of drugs—including the cholesterol-lowering statins, beta-blockers, ACE (angiotensin-converting enzyme) inhibitors, and calcium channel antagonists—has been a boon. So have advances in diagnostic equipment and ever-more-ingenious surgical techniques. Perhaps most exciting, the frontier of gene therapy holds enormous promise, including the possibility of actually growing new blood vessels to bypass coronary artery blockages.

But despite these impressive advances, heart disease is presently winning the battle. It remains the leading killer of both men and women in the United States. Someone has a heart attack in our country every 20 seconds. Beyond the death toll, some 100 million Americans—40 percent of our population—have some sort of cardiovascular problem, from coronary artery disease to hypertension (high blood pressure) or diabetes. Without better tools to prevent heart disease, the future looks even more bleak. Consider these troubling facts.

> ■ *Despite all the evangelism on behalf of low-fat, low-cholesterol diets, one study showed that Americans are, on average, heavier than ever. Obesity is a cardiovascular risk factor.*

> ■ *The federal government, academic medicine, and the pharmaceutical and food industries are all working together, albeit with the best of intentions, to steamroll us with a frightening and untrue message: Fat and cholesterol are bad for you. This misinformation from the medical establishment has achieved so much undeserved credibility that I call it the Fat Machine. I'll provide you with the truth about cholesterol in your diet in chapter 4.*

> ■ *The incidence of heart disease among women is spiking dramatically. No one has quite figured out why, but the fact is indisputable.*

> ■ *The huge baby-boom generation, 70 million strong, is aging right into the clutches of heart disease.*

> ■ *No less an organization than the American Heart Association believes that heart disease and stroke are reaching epidemic levels. Beyond the cost in lives, heart disease is also a tremendous financial burden on our medical system. We already spend $164 billion annually on treatments for heart and blood vessel diseases, and those numbers could explode in the near future as the general population ages.*

Yes, a proper diet is very important. But clearly, it is not enough. Most people who have heart attacks don't have elevated cholesterol levels.

Yes, exercise is important, too. It can help cut your risk of heart disease. But it, too, is not enough. Everybody has a story of a neighbor or co-worker who worked out every day and was nonetheless felled by a heart attack.

Stress reduction matters as well. But we need stronger weapons. The Carnitine Defense is the new nutraceutical hope. The ingredients of the Cardiac Elixir are:

- *Carnitine*
- *Vitamin E*
- *Vitamin B$_6$*
- *Vitamin B$_{12}$*
- *Folic acid*
- *Magnesium*
- *Alcohol*

Those concerned about achieving optimal heart health should consider taking supplements of the first six plus a small to moderate amount of alcohol as part of a cardiovascular health plan.

Choosing Elixir Ingredients

I wrote this book in part because there is a lot of confusion out there about natural substances. People are taking lots of different supplements without much understanding of the medical facts. I thought that I could do a service by describing the state of medical knowledge, explaining exactly what we know about cardiovascular nutraceuticals. Some natural-healing enthusiasts will argue, I'm sure, that the Cardiac Elixir prescription is too narrow. After all, not a day goes by when there isn't some new heart-tonic claim for another natural substance, be it garlic or hawthorn or fish oil or coenzyme Q$_{10}$ or vitamin C. And, to be sure, a great many substances have shown some early potential as having beneficial cardiac properties. I wrestled with the question of which nutraceuticals to include in the Cardiac Elixir. But finally, I elected to limit my recommendations to only those substances that are reasonably validated by clinical studies and supported by expert physicians.

Here's my thinking. Even the best clinical studies can be difficult to interpret. For example, the results of a long-term clinical study revealed that fiber, a nutraceutical that for years had been recommended to help prevent colon cancer, actually did not offer protection against the disease. Experts were confounded because both the original studies that reported fiber as a colon cancer–fighter and the single, better-controlled new one that contradicted it appeared to be well-designed and well-executed. Both studies looked at thousands of people and followed them over many years.

Some skeptics about nutraceuticals will point to this kind of reversal as evidence that oftentimes we're just guessing, that statistics can be manipulated to suggest anything that any scientist with an agenda wants them to. But that attitude is destructive and, more important, completely misses the truth of the matter. This kind of reversal doesn't mean that science is corrupt; quite the opposite— it proves that it's honest. When clinical studies come to different conclusions, it just means that the jury is still out on fiber. It doesn't mean that our research is useless; it just means that clinical research is hard to do, that biological truth is elusive, and that we have to be more ingenious in designing our clinical studies.

My own hunch is that fiber may be proven to help prevent some types of cancer. Indeed, I think that fiber will continue to be shown to help thwart heart disease. But do we have definitive medical proof for either? No, not yet. On fiber, the game's afoot. My feeling is that the cause of nutraceuticals has been hurt, not helped, by common premature healing claims for substances that are based on bad or insufficient data, studies done with too few subjects over too short a period or with too few controls for variables. So I've been conservative in my recommendations. I'm confident that with time, clinical research will discover other nutraceuticals that can protect our hearts. Many doctors who are working the frontier of heart medicine, practicing what is sometimes called complementary cardiology, are already prescribing many other nutraceuticals to short-circuit the pathologies that lead to heart disease. Five years hence, a Cardiac Elixir will surely include substances in addition to those I suggest here. In part three of this book, I discuss some of the substances that almost made it into the mix, including fiber, fish

Talk to Your Doctor about Nutraceuticals

It feels to me as though people are frustrated with their doctors these days. I hear a lot of complaints that people can't get enough of their doctor's time or attention. There's no question that the pressures—financial and otherwise—on doctors have strained the doctor-patient relationship. As a result, some people have taken more responsibility for their own health care. In some respects, this empowerment is all to the good. The wisest patients aren't passive, but actively engaged in their own well-being. The best patients ask the right questions and try to understand their health status. But it's important that you don't get carried away with self-care. As the philosopher Francis Bacon pointed out: "A little learning is a dangerous thing." With the proliferation of medical information, not-always-accurate advice in every newspaper and online, it's easy to go astray and come to think that you know more than you do.

On behalf of all the doctors who believe in nutraceuticals, I implore you to keep these thoughts in mind.

There is no substitute for a good relationship with a doctor. You need access to your doctor's training and experience and should do everything you can to get that access. Don't be shy about asking questions. This is your health you're talking about. Nobody cares about it as much as you do. Be sure that you're tapping all of your doctor's knowledge.

Full disclosure is vital. I am always astonished by statistics about the large number of people who don't tell their doctors everything they need to

oil, coenzyme Q_{10}, niacin, and others. (For more on some of these substances, see chapter 13.)

Of course, you can't discuss preventive medicine without controversy. For every nutraceutical extremist who thinks that I'm a slow-moving dinosaur, there will be somebody who thinks that I'm too bullish on some of these substances. They'll argue that there haven't been definitive clinical studies that definitely prove the cardiac benefits of some of the ingredients of the Cardiac Elixir. They're not exactly wrong. In part because heart disease has know. Many people, for example, don't reveal that they're taking a particular drug or herb or supplement. In the most extreme cases, withholding this kind of information can lead to severe interactions. We are molecular soups, and every addition to our systems changes the mix a bit. To be at his best, your doctor needs to know everything about your health status—both everything you're taking and all of your signs and symptoms as well.

Never take any supplements without your doctor's approval or, at least, knowledge. Though the nutraceuticals in the Cardiac Elixir—carnitine; vitamins E, B_6, and B_{12}; folic acid; magnesium; and alcohol—are safe for most of us, there are people who shouldn't take supplements of one or more of these ingredients. Further, there are certain medical situations where the supplements shouldn't be taken, either. Particularly if you're on medications, for your heart or other illnesses, it's vital that you consult your doctor before making any supplements a regular part of your health regimen.

Never stop taking medications before consulting your doctor. This should go without saying, but apparently it doesn't. Statistics suggest that lots of people just stop taking prescription drugs or fail to take them regularly and don't tell their doctors. Also, remember that, except in rare cases, nutraceuticals are not a substitute for pharmaceuticals. They work along with medications. The pharmaceutical-nutraceutical partnership has arrived in modern medicine and will have a major beneficial effect on the prevention and treatment of many diseases.

many different causes, and in part because it most often develops over many years, even a lifetime, it's tough to design conclusive clinical studies about the effect of any particular preventive measure that we take against it.

Often, I'm with the purists. I like to see the results of gold-standard clinical studies before coming to any medical conclusions. But the plain fact is that we aren't going to have any such clinical studies anytime soon. Nobody is doing them. The reasons for that are various. But the bottom line is that the data in support of these cardiovascular nutraceuticals are convincing. Consider these two facts: (1) There are no definitive clinical studies about the benefits of vitamin E, and (2) approximately 80 percent of all doctors take supplemental doses of this vitamin. That means the majority of physicians in the United States disagree with the purists and are now taking a cardiovascular nutraceutical.

The stakes are very high. After all, lots of people are dying of heart disease every day. Think of the Carnitine Defense as a snapshot of the state of medicine and science now. To be sure, our understanding of our bodies is a work in progress. This particular combination of nutraceuticals is an effective place to start, the first step on the path to natural heart disease prevention and, yes, treatment, by taking supplements of natural substances.

Over the years, popular books have moved the public health ball down the field against heart disease. In the 1960s, Dr. Kenneth Cooper's *Aerobics* endorsed the importance of exercise for cardiovascular health. In the 1970s, *Type A Behavior and Your Heart* by Dr. Meyer Friedman and Dr. Ray Rosenman revealed the importance of anger and stress management. In the 1980s, many books began to promote the low-fat and low-cholesterol dietary approach to preventing heart disease. Dr. Dean Ornish's books have helped make the imperatives of low-fat, low-cholesterol eating pretty close to common knowledge. Though I have some reservations about the Ornish program, which I'll discuss in chapter 4, there's no question that the right approach to diet can be important. But the Carnitine Defense is yet another step in moving the ball of public health down the field in our fight against heart disease.

CHAPTER TWO

Giving Mother Nature a Hand: Why Diet Is Not Enough

Any call for changes in conventional wisdom and fixed social patterns tends to stir people up. On more than a few occasions over the years, I've gotten myself in some trouble by actually saying out loud that diet doesn't matter when it comes to preventing heart disease. When I give talks, it's one of my favorite rabble-rousing first sentences. The diet-doesn't-matter opening never fails to send a slightly hostile murmur through the crowd.

Of course, it's not true.

Diet does matter. Avoiding excessive fat and sugar in your diet is a prudent approach to taking care of your heart and blood vessels. Though I believe that the low-fat evangelism has gone too far (more about that in chapter 4), it's nonetheless clear that a diet loaded with fresh fruits and vegetables is a better health bet than one that is loaded with processed foods high in fat—not just to prevent heart disease but to prevent many other illnesses as well.

If Some Is Good, Is More Better?

The cause of nutraceuticals has been hurt over the years by people who, in my view, take advocacy of supplementation way too far. There are supplementation disciples out there who recommend megadoses of many different natural molecules. They seem to operate on the idea that if some of a substance is good for you, more must be better.

This is muddled thinking. After all, a river can irrigate a field, but a flood destroys the crop. One drink a day may be good for you, but four can be a disaster. There are plenty of situations where you can get too much of a good thing. Indeed, one of the challenges of the nutraceutical revolution is figuring out exactly what the optimum dosage is and at what level we get the most health-protecting bang for our nutraceutical buck. If we can eventually master the mysteries of individual metabolism, we may well be able to find precisely the amount of each food ingredient that each of us needs. If some is good, more might indeed be better—but it might be worse.

Where does that leave us? It's too soon to say. Only clinical research will reveal the answer. The guidelines in this book provide a good starting point, and exceeding them is not advisable until there is more information.

Then why do I say that diet doesn't matter? Because this overstatement helps me get people's attention to make an important point about the overlooked opportunity to fight disease by taking supplements of nutraceuticals.

A healthy diet is important, but clearly, it's not enough. In a way, the success with which the low-fat, low-cholesterol message has been spread has given us tunnel vision and kept us from seeing the much broader benefits in nutraceuticals. Many folks think that if they eat low-fat foods, exercise often, and minimize their stress, they're doing everything they can to cut their risk of heart disease. These prevention strategies have made it into mainstream medicine. They have been endorsed by academic medicine, the government, and the food and drug industries. Nutraceuticals are still on their voyage toward the mainstream. We're so focused on dietary and exercise directives that we've overlooked the preventive power in supplements. I believe that the cardiovascular benefits of supplements dwarf the cardiovascular benefits of the low-fat diets that have been promoted so strongly. Let me repeat: This is not to diminish the importance of diet. A healthy diet is vital. After all, foods are loaded with nutraceuticals. Eating them is a sensible way to get the ingredients of the Cardiac Elixir.

Vitamin E, one component of the Elixir, is present in a variety of foods, including cashews; sunflower seeds; oils, including soybean oil, safflower oil, and corn oil; whole grains; wheat germ; and spinach.

You can feature another component, folic acid, for dinner if you eat pinto beans, navy beans, lentils, okra, black-eyed peas, spinach, or asparagus. To get still another component, vitamin B_6, you should try watermelon, bananas, potatoes, rice, or chicken. Magnesium is part of the Elixir, too, and for food-based magnesium, tofu is a good source. So are kidney beans, chickpeas, peanut butter, artichokes, and halibut.

I urge you to eat a balanced diet and load up on these nutraceutical-rich foods. But don't stop there. There's compelling data to support this central nutraceutical fact: Our bodies can benefit from levels of these nutraceuticals higher than the levels that can be attained through diet.

Clinical studies show that we just can't eat enough of the foods to get certain nutraceuticals to their optimally protective levels. To get the cardiovascular protection available from supplements of vitamin E , you would have to eat 10 cups of peanut butter or 100 cups of spinach every day. To get the benefits available from supplementation with folic acid, you'd have to gorge on 3 cups of dried figs or 9 oranges. To get the benefits of supplemental magnesium, you'd have to devour 2 cups of brown rice or 16 servings of beets.

Even if you could eat all this food, the calories that come with it would probably make you put on weight. By taking supplements of nutraceuticals, you get the biochemical armor without the calories that you don't need.

Carnitine, the centerpiece of the Cardiac Elixir, is found primarily in meats and dairy products. To get the carnitine heart protection available from supplementation, you'd have to eat more steaks per day than even an NFL linebacker could manage. Even if you could do it, steaks also come with fat and cholesterol that at excessive levels are bad for you. Supplementation with carnitine tablets or capsules lets you, as the old song says, accentuate the positive and eliminate the negative.

RDAs and the Uniqueness of You

I want to talk a little about RDAs, or Recommended Dietary Allowances. These are the guidelines developed by the National Research Council for how much of various nutrients that you need to stay healthy. Many will argue that these levels are just fine. I disagree. In general, I think that they're way too low. In making a decision about taking supplements, keep in mind these thoughts about the limitations of RDAs.

They're not very ambitious for our health. RDAs were developed to meet certain nutritional needs, not take advantage of health opportunities. Given the tremendous optimal health possibilities of the nutraceutical revolution, it makes no sense to base a nutritional program on such modest goals. Why settle for "healthy enough" when you can enhance and protect your well-being far beyond that level? In fact, many nutraceuticals do not even have RDAs.

They can't account for particular risk factors. Even healthy people are at greater risk for some illnesses than others. For example, if you have risk factors for heart disease—a family history, a weight problem, high blood lipid levels, a stressful life—you surely can benefit from higher levels of cardiovascular nutraceuticals than people who have no risk factors.

Drugs May Make Supplements Necessary

You probably already know that some drugs interact with others, either magnifying or masking their potency. But did you know that they can also react with nutrients and prevent our bodies from using the nutrients optimally?

It's true. If you take particular prescription or over-the-counter medications at the same time you take your supplements, your body may not be able to fully absorb good stuff like vitamin E, B vitamins, or magnesium. Worse, some medications can even leach these important nutrients from your body.

To prevent deficiencies, check with your doctor or pharmacist about possible interactions of the prescription and over-the-counter drugs you take. Also, always follow your doctor's instructions about when to take your medication.

Here are some common medications along with which heart-healthy supplements they may destroy.

Medication	May Affect Availability of
Antacids	Folate
Antibacterial agents	Vitamin B_6, folate
Antibiotics	Magnesium, potassium
Anti-cancer drugs	Magnesium, folate
Antihypertensives	Vitamin B_6
Anti-inflammatories	Folate, vitamin B_{12}
Diuretics	Magnesium, potassium, folate
Cholesterol-lowering drugs	Folate, vitamin B_{12}

If you're a smoker or lead a high-stress life, the nutrient levels in RDAs probably won't even meet your requirements for minimal health. These lifestyle factors make you use up some nutrients just dealing with toxic effects of heavy cigarette smoke or stress-related chemicals.

They're based on statistical averages and norms, and you're probably not average. Remember the old warning about putting your trust in averages: If it floods one day and is dry the next, an average rainfall doesn't tell you much about the local weather.

Now granted, the RDAs are based on very broad samples, so they're not without usefulness. But it's important to understand that you have your own unique biochemistry. You may require far more or less of a certain nutrient than your next-door neighbor. Indeed, some people need 10 times as much of certain nutrients as others do.

They're based on the needs of healthy people. You may be sick and not know it. The heart cells of people who have myocardial ischemia, for instance—medical terminology for lack of oxygen to the heart, usually caused by a blockage of blood to the heart—are deficient in carnitine. But their blood levels of carnitine, and the levels of carnitine in the areas of their heart with a normal blood supply, are normal.

Heart disease deprives your heart of carnitine where it needs this substance most. Even if you were tested for carnitine levels, your blood level of carnitine could be normal. Nonetheless, you need supplementation.

Each of us is a unique biological system with our own metabolic story. Some of us utilize one vitamin poorly and another mineral quite efficiently. So we may need higher-than-average doses of the nutrients that we don't handle well and lower-than-average amounts of those that our systems handle efficiently. My point is that a blood test might show you to be within a "normal" range for magnesium or potassium or zinc, and yet, in terms of your particular metabolic requirements, you could be deficient. Any deficiency can compromise many different biological processes and put you at risk for many diseases.

To be sure, there are some nutrients that you can get too much of. Since many nutraceuticals interact, a high level of one may throw off the balance required for proper interaction. So before you start taking any supplement, you should talk with your doctor.

Diets and Discipline: We're Human, Not Animals in Cages

When considering your health, it's important to be truthful to yourself. Most of us love food that doesn't exactly fall in the low-fat category. We like a nice steak now and then. Most of us are also enthusiasts when it comes to food. Dietary discipline is not easy.

Sound familiar? Ever have trouble resisting ice cream on a summer afternoon? Or a doughnut to go with your morning coffee? Of course you do. You're a human being, and those foods are tempting. After all, we're all children of Eve, and she fell for a plain old apple. Any wonder that a Philadelphia cheesesteak is pretty alluring?

The evidence is clear. Despite all the publicity about the importance of eating well, we're just not doing it. One study showed that, on average, we're heavier than ever. We know that we should eat more fruits and vegetables, but most of us aren't doing it.

Why? There are lots of reasons, including the fact that meal preparation often gets lost in the whirl of hectic lives. We eat on the fly, and we eat packaged, processed, nutritionally deficient foods because they're convenient. But behind all the sociological explanations is a simple fact: We like the taste of high-fat foods, and we find it understandably difficult to resist them.

Sure, we should eat three to five servings of fruits and vegetables every day. And we should be loyal friends and perfect parents. And we should work hard and save our money and floss every day. But we're flawed, and we're subservient to our tastebuds.

The same situation applies to exercise. Everybody knows that we should move our bodies more. The data convincingly show that physically active people have healthier hearts than sedentary folks. But many of us don't want to go out jogging or lift weights; we want to stay inside where it's nice and warm and watch the ball game.

Estimates are that four out of five Americans are not physically active enough to get the full health benefits of exercise. I exercise because I enjoy it, and I believe that it keeps me well. But let's face it—many others don't enjoy it and simply won't exercise. As a physician, I believe that it's important to face the reality of people's lives. We do our patients no service if we just keep giving them advice they're not going to follow. We keep shouting "diet and exercise, diet and exercise," and people are getting heart disease in unprecedented numbers. We have to hear the harsh truth that the diet-and-exercise approach to preventing heart disease has failed.

One of the many benefits of supplementation for cardiac health is that it doesn't require much discipline. Taking supplements is especially important for people who find it tough to stick to low-fat diets and make themselves exercise.

Over the years, some of my critics have accused me of offering people a quick fix, of promoting "health in a bottle." My editor says that it's unfair to claim that people who disagree with me are under the sway of some prejudice that is distorting their judgment. But here goes, anyway.

I believe that many critics of supplementation have a quasi-religious attachment to the idea that we need only eat at Mother Nature's bountiful table to get all the nutrients that we need. Somehow, the idea of taking a nutraceutical pill smacks of high-tech, of being unnatural. It isn't. It's a celebration of both Mother Nature and human nature—the molecules that keep us well and the ingenuity that it took for our species to figure it out.

The data on behalf of supplementation are strong. For the record, I do not see supplements as a replacement for good dietary habits. But they are an essential companion to them. Supplements can help you stay healthier, particularly if you lack the willingness or ability to watch what you eat.

CHAPTER THREE

Beyond Capitalism and Cure

A few years ago, the *New York Times* ran a profile of me under the headline "The Don Quixote of Nutraceuticals." I wasn't sure if I was delighted or dismayed. On one hand, Cervantes' hero, the Spanish knight who tilted at windmills, is a defender of truth, justice, and good causes.

But clearly, the name *Don Quixote* also carries with it a connotation of hopelessness. It can be used to describe a person whose fight is foolish and futile despite determination and good intentions.

For the record, over the course of my career, in my efforts to promote the medical benefits of natural substances, I have indeed tilted at my share of windmills. I have run into a great deal of opposition and, even more disturbingly, indifference. The road to public acceptance of nutraceuticals has been quite rocky. In a way, one of the great breakthroughs in modern chemistry is to blame.

Magic Bullets and Big Money

Almost 100 years ago, the great German bacteriologist Paul Ehrlich developed a way to treat syphilis with an arsenic compound. Ehrlich's work was a big step against a disease that, at the time, was common and often fatal. The treatment itself— Ehrlich called the medicine Salvarsan—was important. But in a way, the phrase that Ehrlich used to describe it was even more influential.

Magic bullet.

The phrase had a wonderful dramatic ring to it, evoking images of both alchemy and battle. Ehrlich's breakthrough against syphilis and his powerful metaphor—that chemicals could be fired at disease—became the engine of medical research. Scientists went in search of magic bullets—single substances, not mixtures—that could conquer disease without harming the patient.

By the 1920s, Frederick Banting, M.D., and Charles Best, M.D., of the University of Toronto, Ontario, had discovered that insulin was a magic bullet against diabetes. The antibiotics developed in the 1940s were magic bullets against infection. Many medical milestones grew from this idea.

Something else grew out of it as well: the pharmaceutical industry. The genius of capitalism seized on the business opportunity in the magic bullet idea.

How did this work against the emergence of nutraceuticals? Simple. Drugs, which are primarily artificial molecules, were so successful, both as medicines and as business ventures, that they became a juggernaut, overwhelming the huge medical promise of natural substances.

It's difficult to get strong patent protection on a natural substance. Once you get past all the legal details, the rule is pretty simple: If God came up with the molecule, you can't claim it and sell it exclusively. So any company selling a natural substance, be it garlic or vitamin E or spring water or carnitine, is probably going to have lots of competition from other companies. Artificial molecules, on the other hand, can be protected by a strong patent for up to 20 years. So, once a Pfizer gets a patent and FDA approval for a drug like Viagra, it can sell that substance exclusively for a long time and realize billions of dollars in revenue. As you can see, a successful drug for a common health problem, like arthritis, depression, or high blood pressure, can be a financial bonanza for pharmaceutical companies.

The important point is that there's little financial incentive for big drug companies to invest the large amounts of capital required to do research into the preventive and therapeutic effects of carnitine, folate, magnesium, or any other natural substance. Once they do, competing companies can then swoop in and, most often, since they haven't spent any money on the research, sell the substance at lower cost.

Back when I was just beginning my clinical research into carnitine, like a lot of physicians, I was scrambling for funding. So, armed with what I considered impressive preliminary data, I naively approached some colleagues in the pharmaceutical industry. I got a quick lesson in how medicine and money are intertwined. The drug people were cordial, even intrigued by my results. But they were not about to invest in studying carnitine.

Why? Since carnitine is a natural substance, it can't be protected by a strong patent. I can't tell you how many times over the years I've heard someone from a drug company say some variation of, "It's financial suicide for us; we just can't do it" when I tried to encourage investment in research on carnitine or another nutraceutical that had shown clear medicinal promise.

I don't mean this as a knock on the drug companies. I'm not describing a conspiracy or any deliberate attempt by an evil medical empire to keep powerful medicines from the people. For the most part, I admire the scientists, doctors, and drug company professionals I've worked with over the years. Can you imagine a world without antibiotics, vaccines, and other pharmaceuticals? After all, corporate executives are entitled, even obliged, to make sound business judgments. The plain fact is that they're just not in the business of doing research on nutraceutical substances.

There's no question in my mind that the enormous success of our drug companies has, along with powerful government disincentives that raise the cost of basic and clinical research tremendously, inhibited the growth of natural medicines that may be both safer and less expensive than drugs. Estimates indicate that the total cost to obtain just one FDA-approved drug is more than $500 million! Keep in mind that not only do drug companies have little interest in researching nutraceuticals but they also have a powerful vested interest in promoting unnatural ones. Powerful marketing campaigns on behalf of the magic bullets have made us—both doctors and patients—drug-dependent.

I don't mean that we're addicted to drugs in the biological sense of the word, but just that drugs are often the first line of therapy that both patients and physicians think of when we're sick, whether we get a serious illness or a summer cold. We've become habituated to managing disease through pharmaceuticals rather than preventing or treating it with nutraceuticals.

I worry that we take drugs with too little thought about possible alternatives. As patients, we lack patience. When we go to the doctor, we're not looking for a dietary or supplement program that will make us well. No, we want the quick fix, the magic bullet that will get us back in the game as soon as possible. Often, we tend to think pharmaceutically about cure when we should be thinking nutraceutically about prevention.

Breaking Through the Culture of Cure

In much the same way that the success of artificial molecules—drugs—has stolen the thunder of nature's nutraceutical molecules, the effort to cure disease has overwhelmed the effort to prevent it. Don't misunderstand me. My official position is that

I'm all for curing disease. Indeed, the curing achievements of medical researchers and drug companies are one of the great stories of the modern era. Dozens of diseases that used to kill millions have been all but eradicated because smart scientists and physicians put them in the crosshairs and set out to find a magic bullet against them.

But precisely because cure is such a good story, medical research has developed in a one-dimensional way. There's no question that the emphasis has been on beating disease rather than on enhancing health to prevent disease. The cure-disease model has become the 500-pound gorilla, shoving the prevent-disease model offstage into the wings.

One of the reasons why it's tough to get funding for research into preventive medicine is because it's just not a good story. Over the years, many writers and editors have said that they can't run headlines that say something like "Ten Million People Don't Get Heart Disease." Something that is not happening is not a story. Nutraceuticals, which keep us from getting sick, don't have a media hook. They only keep catastrophe from happening.

Inevitably, money for research tends to flow toward science that gets media coverage. And government funding, one of the few sources of money other than drug companies, tends to go toward research aimed at cures, in part because specific diseases like AIDS or breast cancer have advocacy groups working in their behalf. Of course, I'm not arguing that we stop looking for cures, but we need some balance.

In 1976, I started the Foundation for Innovation in Medicine (FIM). My mission was to raise money for research into nutraceuticals and tip the seesaw a little more toward prevention. In a way, I thought of myself as a lobbyist for Mother Nature. For a time, I worked without much success, tilting at the twin windmills: the uninterested pharmaceutical industry and the media. I was beginning to lose faith, when one of nature's medicines broke through, leaping from obscurity into prominence and starting the nutraceutical revolution.

The Big Bang of Nutraceuticals

Just as physicists believe that the universe began at a certain moment with a great big bang, the nutraceutical revolution started with a similar singular event. In 1983, the National Institutes of Health convened a group of medical experts to assess the role of calcium supplementation for the prevention and management of osteoporosis. The expert physicians concluded that supplemental calcium could be helpful in preventing postmenopausal bone loss, or osteoporosis. The press picked up the story, and the calcium news spread quickly. Within a month after the conference, it seemed as though everybody had heard about calcium, the first bona fide modern nutraceutical.

All these years later, I still don't know exactly why the calcium news exploded the way it did. There had been plenty of clinical evidence on behalf of nutraceuticals before then. Perhaps the old Eastern wisdom is right: When the student is ready, the teacher will arrive. But it was as if some submerged desire to embrace nature's good news had been suddenly released. The big bang of calcium gave birth to the nutraceutical universe. The public appeared ready to accept that, for some health problems, diet was just not enough. Many postmenopausal women just couldn't get the optimum calcium benefit from the food they ate. There was additional protection from osteoporosis available in a supplemental dose of calcium.

I was greatly encouraged by calcium's big media moment. Optimist that I am, I was convinced that the story of nutraceuticals was about to explode into people's health consciousness. But it didn't happen, at least not right away. For a time, it looked as though calcium would be a uniquely famous nutraceutical. But then, two other nutraceuticals got their big breaks, too. Fiber and fish oil made some health headlines as well. Physicians announced that supplements of fiber could help prevent colon cancer, and supplements of fish oil could work to thwart heart disease. Though subsequent studies would show that the data on fiber and fish oil were shaky, these announcements were nonetheless important indicators.

Just like the calcium news, the fiber and fish oil news spread quickly through the media. It was now clear that people were enthused about the nutraceutical message, open to the idea that supplements of natural substances could keep them well.

Over the past decade, many other natural substances—vitamin C, beta-carotene, vitamin E, and melatonin, to name just a few—have had their time in the media sun. In fact, at the risk of sounding like a malcontent, I'm tempted to complain that the media pendulum has now swung too far *toward* "unproven" natural remedies. A lot of the media coverage of nutraceuticals is way out ahead of medicine, announcing "miracles" based on small or poorly designed studies. But given my choice between too much coverage and the vacuum of too little, in which nutraceuticals languished for so long, I'll take the former.

At this point, nutraceuticals are not recommended as a replacement for pharmaceuticals. They're another tool, an additional wellness weapon. Before describing the pathology of heart disease, and exactly how each of the ingredients in the Cardiac Elixir works, I think it's important to explain a few nutraceutical principles to show how these natural weapons work against disease to keep you well.

Beyond Magic and Bullets: Some New Ways of Thinking

Like a lot of physicians, I have a vivid memory of the first moment I thought about studying medicine. I was 9 years old when my grandmother fell into a diabetic coma. Back then, dying was different than it is now. My grandmother wasn't rushed to the hospital. Instead, my parents put a bed in the dining room so we could watch over her. I remember one night, just watching my grandmother lie there and thinking one of those boyish thoughts, that if I could just move something in her brain a little, she'd be okay.

Looking back, I know two things. First, brain jiggling wouldn't have helped my grandmother, and second, nutraceuticals would have. They wouldn't have helped her as much once she was acutely ill, but if she had taken nutraceutical supplements over the years, she probably would have enjoyed more healthy years with fewer tears.

Nutraceuticals could have done the same for my father. He died much too soon of complications from extensive atherosclerosis. Back then, we didn't know that supplements of carnitine could help nourish your heart, that vitamin E could help keep blood vessels resilient, or that folate could help control homocysteine levels. I'm certain that if my father had begun to take the Cardiac Elixir at an earlier age, his life, too, would have been both longer and more enjoyable.

Nutraceuticals work in teams. I've often said that a meal is the perfect metaphor for how nutraceuticals work—a little of this, a little of that. Nature works in mixtures and combinations. So it only makes sense that healing substances would work in mixtures and combinations as well. The calcium from one food works with the magnesium from another. And yet, much of our entire scientific and medical system resists the idea of combination solutions. The very nature of experimental science requires that we isolate a substance and control for variables. This is not a critique of the scientific method, but just to say that nature is subtler than our minds. It's tremendously difficult to assess how substances work in combination in both healthy and sick people.

Each ingredient of the Cardiac Elixir is just part of a heart disease prevention strategy and works on a different piece of the cardiac pathology. Carnitine helps protect the heart itself. Vitamin E and folic acid help protect the arteries. Magnesium helps protect both the heart and the arteries. It's not fully appreciated that natural substances must work in teams. Since heart disease is caused by many factors, the key to protecting yourself against it is thwarting the disease process at each source. No known single substance can do this.

Nutraceuticals have a more-than-additive effect. When it comes to nutraceuticals, one plus one equals more than two. The effect of a combination of nutraceuticals may exceed the impact that you might expect if you simply added up the activity of each individual component. So the health edge that you get from taking carnitine, vitamin E, and folate could be greater than mere addition would suggest.

Nutraceuticals have a broader effect than pharmaceuticals. It's accurate, if oversimplified, to say that pharmaceuticals tend to be more targeted than nutraceuticals. They're designed for this. You take a pill, and because it has been ingeniously engineered by scientists, it zips right to the site of an infection or goes to work against the specific pathologies that may be causing your disease. Nutraceuticals can do this as well, but they can also do many other things. They're not narrowly aimed, like magic bullets. Instead they suffuse throughout the body, enhancing many metabolic processes as they do. This explains why I recommend many nutraceutical combinations to prevent or treat many diseases. It makes sense, and it's good medicine.

Here are just a few examples of the multiple functions of nutraceuticals:

Vitamin C. Humans deprived of vitamin C will eventually come down with a debilitating disease called scurvy, which for centuries cursed sailors on long sea voyages with bleeding gums and body bruises. It was only when the eighteenth-century British explorer Captain James Cook started giving his sailors vitamin C–rich lime juice during their long voyages that crews could avoid the disease completely. Vitamin C is also essential for the manufacture of the protein collagen; it assists in immune function, and it helps manufacture a number of vital hormones.

Calcium. Most people know that calcium plays a vital role in building and maintaining healthy bones and teeth. But this mineral is also essential in helping your muscles contract and your blood clot.

Magnesium. An ingredient in the Cardiac Elixir, magnesium has a kaleidoscope of chameleon-like properties. It is able to activate or stabilize more than 300 completely different enzyme reactions. And it's part of my Elixir because many of these reactions are critical to heart health. Your heart muscle cells need magnesium for every single contraction, your blood vessels need magnesium to stay relaxed and open, your blood itself needs magnesium to clot normally, and most cells in your body need magnesium to access nutrition in the form of glucose. We'll examine magnesium more closely in chapter 10.

Folic acid. Folic acid is one of the B vitamins and another ingredient in the Cardiac Elixir. It can protect your heart by reducing the levels of a substance called homocysteine in your blood. But your blood cells also need it for cell division, and it's critical for healthy nervous system development in fetuses. In fact, doctors recommend that pregnant women supplement with folic acid to prevent neural tube defects, such as spina bifida, in their newborns.

Nutraceuticals play a special role in disease prevention. By taking nutraceuticals when you're well, you can get to root causes of diseases instead of just treating signs and symptoms once a disease process has taken hold. After all, how do you protect your investment in your house? You put on a new roof before the old one starts leaking. You repoint the brickwork before the mortar crumbles. Taking supplements of nutraceuticals is that kind of medicinal care, that kind of stewardship of your body.

These Ounces of Prevention Can Enrich Our Lives

I have spent more than 35 years working at the crossroads of medicine, business, and government, trying to encourage more clinical research on nutraceuticals. For many of those years, I wasn't overly hopeful. There was powerful resistance. But now, things have changed radically. Over the past decade, the nutraceutical message—that supplementation can enhance nature's disease prevention and treatment capacity—has rapidly made its way into hearts and minds, both in the medical community and in general.

I believe that we're on the edge of an exciting, brave new nutraceutical world, that we'll gradually decode the medicinal properties in thousands of natural substances and figure out how to use them to keep ourselves well. Dramatic advances in our understanding of how our bodies work will multiply the impact of that knowledge.

For example, the human genome project, which aspires to identify every one of the tens of thousands of genes in human DNA, will not only tell us who is at special risk for what diseases but may well reveal the secrets of individual metabolism. If we understand the unique chemistry of each individual, we may be able to devise recipes of nutraceutical supplements customized to biochemical eccentricities.

There will be one Elixir of supplements for the man who has a family history of heart disease, a different blend of natural substances for the woman who struggles with depression, yet another combination for the child who gets migraines, and another for the grandmother who is dealing with diabetes. I believe that knowledge of natural substances combined with knowledge of individual metabolism will ultimately help us prevent lots of disease and manage a great deal of what we cannot prevent. Often, these nutraceuticals will be given along with appropriate pharmaceuticals in order to maximize and strengthen their impact on disease.

I often think of a conversation that I had with a researcher who was studying Alzheimer's disease. He told me that he tried not to think of his work as only searching for a cure, but rather as looking for a way to put the disease off until after people had already died of something else. I don't mean to sound flippant, but the idea of disease postponement makes a lot of sense, especially when it comes to heart disease. After all, if we live long enough, most of us will eventually experience some cardiovascular trouble. Heart disease is truly more tragic when it arrives too early, when lives are claimed or diminished prematurely by the onset of avoidable disease.

The tremendous promise of nutraceuticals is that they can keep us healthier longer. In fact, I believe that medicine will one day prove them to be effective against most diseases—major and even minor—within the next quarter-century. I can assure you that I, personally, am counting on it.

CHAPTER FOUR

Diet, Fat, and Cholesterol: Only Half the Heart Health Story

"Every man should eat and drink, and enjoy the good of all his labor."
—*Ecclesiastes*

Warning: The Fat Machine may be hazardous to your health.

And what exactly is the Fat Machine? It has no gears, pulleys, or levers. It doesn't slice, dice, or shred. But it has many parts and is well-oiled. The Fat Machine, as I call it, is actually a powerful collaborative effort on the part of the federal government, academic medicine, and the pharmaceutical and food industries. This "machine" cranks out a monolithic, fear-provoking message: Fat and cholesterol are bad.

The people who operate this machinery are generally honest and competent. Most of them truly believe that all of what they are saying will help a majority of people.

There's just one problem. I happen to think that they're only telling one side of the story. They continuously and unconsciously fail to send another equally important message: *Most people who have heart attacks do not have high cholesterol.* They ignore an elemental truth: *There are other ways in which to reduce heart attacks due to coronary heart disease.*

Don't get me wrong—diet, fat, and cholesterol are important factors in health. The medical science supporting this notion is impressive and convincing. In fact, these are some of the best documented connections in medicine.

Unfortunately, the Fat Machine has spewed out this single message over and over again for more than two decades—a message that the media has obligingly passed on to all of us. Think about it. Hardly a day goes by without a story in the newspapers about cholesterol, a magazine article promoting low-fat foods, or the author of a new diet book appearing on television touting a new surefire weight-loss program.

The result of this single-minded approach, I fear, has led to a rapid increase in cardiovascular disease in many Americans. We are inundated with information on various aspects of diet and nutrition. Yet we have very little understanding of how these important factors fit into a comprehensive health plan to preserve the integrity of our hearts. In short, I believe that the Fat Machine has done more harm than good. Why? Well, that's the tale of this chapter.

In the Beginning

The blueprint for what later became the Fat Machine was drawn in the late 1970s. That's when the National Institutes of Health (NIH) began a campaign to educate all Americans about the cardiovascular risks of high blood cholesterol levels. The message was aggressively promoted and quickly embraced by physicians, the media, and the public. From that moment, the Fat Machine took form.

But like all information tools, the Fat Machine is only as good

DIET, FAT, AND CHOLESTEROL

as the materials fed into it. And in this case, the materials were flawed. You see, the clinical studies to support the evil-cholesterol message, though suggestive, were not at all definitive. Yet the federal government sounded the alarm before the definitive clinical data were in. The pharmaceutical industry, in its effort to promote multibillion-dollar cholesterol-lowering drugs, virtually indoctrinated both physicians and patients. The food industry, without conducting many clinical studies on their particular low-fat products, joined the pharmaceutical industry and the federal government in this fear campaign. Today, I hardly know any physician, academic or practicing, who does not believe in this message. Today, cholesterol and fat continue to hold center stage, and all other messages about preventing heart disease can't find the light of day. Today, if a physician challenges—or even simply questions—the importance of cholesterol in heart disease, one faces professional loss of credibility or even banishment, usually by shunning.

I'll accept that risk. For the truth is, controlling fat and cholesterol through your diet helps, but that is not the entire story. You can be lulled into a false sense of security if you believe that watching your diet is all you need to do to reduce your risk of heart disease. Let's take a closer look at the Fat Machine's message piece by piece.

The Fat Machine's Mantra

As you probably know—if you've been listening to the Fat Machine—cholesterol has been intimately linked to the development of atherosclerosis, the major cause of coronary heart disease and heart attacks. In fact, some physician experts believe that every reduction of cholesterol by 1 percent brings about a 2 percent reduction in heart attack risk. That can be particularly significant for those with high blood concentrations of this soft, waxy fatlike substance.

What you may not know is that your body actually needs cholesterol to help make bile, hormones, and vitamin D. And you also may not know that even if you had no cholesterol at all in your diet, your body would still make all the cholesterol that you need. In fact, your liver produces about 2,000 milligrams of cholesterol a day. So the cholesterol that most people consume in their diets represents just a fraction of the cholesterol in their bodies. The average American male, for instance, consumes about 320 milligrams of cholesterol a day from various animal products such as meat, eggs, milk, and cheese. An average American woman eats about 265 milligrams. That may not sound like much, but once it is absorbed into the body and added to the blood cholesterol produced by your liver, this dietary cholesterol, if consumed in significant amounts, can have a devastating impact on the cardiovascular health of certain (though not all) people.

Of course, like many substances in the body, cholesterol is complex. So for simplicity, the Fat Machine has divided cholesterol into two categories of lipoproteins, the protein-coated substances that help transport cholesterol through the blood. These categories play a big role in current thinking on cholesterol.

High-density lipoproteins (HDLs). These help the body remove cholesterol by carrying it away from the arteries to the liver where it is excreted. In lay language, HDLs are called the good cholesterol. The evidence we have suggests that a higher level of HDLs lowers your risk of developing heart disease.

Low-density lipoproteins (LDLs). These can cause problems. They help deposit cholesterol in the walls of your arteries. This can lead to clogging of the arteries, the development of atherosclerosis, and later, heart disease. LDLs are the so-called bad cholesterol. When you go to your doctor to have your blood cholesterol levels measured, the number you get refers to your total cholesterol.

What levels of total cholesterol, HDLs, and LDLs indicate that you are in good health as far as these measures are concerned? There is great disagreement over this, and the numbers keep changing. Some extremists are now recommending a cholesterol level of 150 milligrams per deciliter (mg/dl), but current thinking by the experts is that a total cholesterol level of 200 mg/dl should be the dividing line. The higher your level is above that, the greater the increase in your risk of developing heart disease. Conversely, the lower the level of cholesterol, the lower the risk of developing heart disease.

If you're healthy and have no risk factors for heart disease, then an LDL level under 130 mg/dl is considered good. If you have symptoms of heart disease, then an LDL level under 100 mg/dl is considered good. If you have an LDL reading between 130 and 160 mg/dl, your doctor may advise you to watch what you eat. If your LDL level is over 160 mg/dl, you may be asked to consider taking cholesterol-lowering drugs.

With HDLs, Fat Machine experts say the more the merrier. High levels are considered good for your arteries. An HDL level under 35 mg/dl is too low. In addition, the ratio between your total cholesterol level and your HDL level is an important predictor in terms of heart disease. For example, if you had a total blood cholesterol level of 200 mg/dl, and an HDL level of 50 mg/dl, you would divide 200 by 50 to find your ratio, which would be 4. The optimal number here is 3.5; any number higher than that suggests an increased risk of heart disease. These cholesterol numbers are only estimates, based on suggestive—and not definitive—clinical studies.

Fat's Well-Worn Story

Despite all the negative associations with the word, fat is actually an extremely important nutrient. It is used by your body to create energy, and it helps the body absorb many vitamins. Fat and cholesterol are closely related. The amount of fats in your diet influences the amount of cholesterol in your body. Just as there are good cholesterol and bad cholesterol, there are good fats and bad fats.

Saturated fats. This kind of fat can help raise your blood cholesterol levels significantly. Meats and high-fat dairy products are common sources of saturated fats. Foods with saturated fats in them are easily recognized—they are solid at room temperature. Remember, though, that saturated fats are not bad in and of themselves. It's the amount consumed, along with other dietary habits, that may have a bad effect.

Unsaturated fats. These fats are found in plant oils and are liquid at room temperature. They are less likely to raise your cholesterol levels. However, some believe that you can have too much unsaturated fat in your diet as well. Today, experts recommend that fats make up no more than 30 percent of your total daily intake of calories. And unsaturated fats should make up most of that fat consumption. The Fat Machine believes that a low-fat diet helps lower your risk of developing heart disease.

The Other Side of Cholesterol

The Fat Machine's message is a fine one—as far as it goes. It simply doesn't go far enough. And even though medical evidence backs up many of its claims, there are still enough kinks in the machinery to cast reasonable doubt on some of its presumptions.

Take cholesterol, for instance. Even after all these years, there still isn't convincing clinical evidence that lowering cholesterol by eating low-fat foods, either natural or artificial, will significantly reduce heart attacks. It may turn out to be true, but the clinical evidence is simply not there now.

Certainly, there is unequivocal evidence from pharmaceutical trials demonstrating that lowering cholesterol levels by use of drugs will prevent heart attacks. But, in its zeal, the Fat Machine is dangerously close to running amok with these drugs.

The clinical trials that deal with heart disease usually involve administering the cholesterol-lowering drug over a limited period of time, for example, 5 years, and measuring the number of heart attacks during this time. Because of improvements in public hygiene and the miracles of modern medicine, we are generally living for a much longer period of time than in the recent past. No one questions that cholesterol-lowering drugs are powerful chemicals that interfere with natural metabolic pathways. The good news is that these drugs appear to save lives over a 5-year period.

But what happens when people who are living longer continue to take these pills over the next 20 to 30 years? We don't know. The evidence is not in yet. But the question remains as to whether the human body can tolerate such powerful drugs over long periods of time. In a disturbing development, there is now an effort to promote the use of these drugs not only among those with high cholesterol levels but also among people with normal cholesterol levels. It is not inconceivable that 50 percent of the U.S. adult population will be on cholesterol-lowering drugs in the near future without a reasonable assessment of the potential toxicity that may occur with long-term consumption.

This, in my opinion, could lead to a national tragedy. Indeed, the cholesterol-lowering message pushed by the Fat Machine is so powerful that there are now serious attempts to severely restrict dietary fat intake among children in an attempt to accommodate this overrated belief. This effort clearly involves experimentation with children that could severely impair their physical and mental development.

But is anyone objecting? Not many. Physicians, parents, and educators think that this is okay because they have been indoctrinated by the Fat Machine into believing that the evils of fat and cholesterol threaten the health of America's children. If a physician were to perform a clinical trial to determine whether a psycho-stimulant drug could help kids with mental problems, there likely would be an overwhelming negative public reaction fueled by the mass media. Yet silence greets a massive experiment that is beginning to be conducted on our children at the urging of the Fat Machine. While I have no quarrel with improving the dietary habits of children, it's how we do it that concerns me.

Obesity: Bigger, Not Better

There is little doubt that the Fat Machine's efforts to educate the public about the detrimental effects of excessive fat consumption on the heart has had a major beneficial impact. This effort has helped reduce cardiovascular disease in a large segment of the population. On the other hand, I fear that this attempt has paradoxically led to an increase in heart disease in another significant segment of our population—the obese.

Obesity can be defined as the excessive accumulation of body fat. Though there are many exceptions to the numbers given, there are standard height-weight tables that you can use to determine if you are in the weight range from normal to obese. Somewhat arbitrarily, a person who is 20 percent over what these tables list as normal is considered obese.

With each passing decade, the U.S. population becomes more obese. At the beginning of the 1990s, it was estimated that 24 percent of American men and 27 percent of American women were obese. As we enter the twenty-first century, those figures have risen to 30 percent for both men and women. Obesity has more than doubled among Americans between the ages of 20 and 55. There is little doubt that there is a severe obesity epidemic in our country.

So what does all this have to do with the Fat Machine's obsession with low-fat eating? I'm going to let you in on a little secret: The rise in obesity in the United States parallels the rise in the popularity of low-fat diets. The problem is many Americans have failed to recognize that low-fat or fat-free foods are still loaded with calories, mainly carbohydrates. In fact, some fat-free products have more calories than the original. Even if a low-fat product doesn't have more calories per serving, some people may be more tempted to eat a whole bag or box of snack food because they don't realize that excess calories are converted into fat.

So it is not unreasonable to assume that our emphasis on

low-fat foods has boomeranged and is one of the major factors in bringing about our current U.S. obesity epidemic. And, as we all know, obesity itself is a major cause of cardiovascular disease ranging from hypertension (high blood pressure) to heart attacks.

The Ornish Studies on Low-Fat Eating

Let's look at one celebrated study conducted by famed physician Dean Ornish, M.D., whose research about reversing heart disease is extremely popular but also somewhat controversial. Dr. Ornish wanted to test the hypothesis that diet, along with changes in lifestyle, can retard or even reverse the growth of a coronary artery plaque. He placed patients on a very low fat diet, one to which few could adhere over a long period of time. His studies, published in the *Journal of the American Medical Association*, or *JAMA*, reported that patients on his diet had slightly wider coronary arteries and a significant reduction in chest pain.

Having been prepared for years by the Fat Machine, the mass media trumpeted the results of this study to both professionals and the public. Many of my physician colleagues fervently embraced the media's message and recommend very low fat diets to their patients. After all, the reasoning was medically sound. Publication in *JAMA* usually means that the study was well-conducted and that the conclusions are believable. However, in this case, people were just waiting for this message to be born, and they embraced it wholeheartedly.

Unfortunately, the study is simply too limited in scope to accept it as the final word. Gina Kolata of *The New York Times*, one of the nation's premier medical writers, interviewed a few major cardiovascular experts regarding Dr. Ornish's study. In their view, though the message is highly attractive, too few patients were evaluated to make any definitive, positive conclusions. This, by the way, is in line with my own thinking and that of some of my colleagues.

Paul D. Thompson, M.D., the director of preventive cardiology at Harvard Hospital stated, "Rarely have so many conclusions been based on so few subjects."

Frank Sacks, M.D., a nutrition expert and professor at the Harvard School of Public Health, noted that there was no improvement in the size of the coronary arteries in the more narrowed parts, the parts in which blood clots and blockage are most likely to occur and to lead to heart attacks.

Robert Eckel, M.D., professor of medicine at the University of Colorado Health Science Center in Denver, stated that to measure such an effect would require a study involving thousands of patients for a period of years.

Dr. Ornish deserves credit and congratulations for his creative attempt to demonstrate how a low-fat diet can reduce the severity of coronary artery disease. We must, however, await the results of future published clinical studies to confirm his conclusions before we accept this reasonable assumption.

Frankly, many people recommend low-fat diets, despite the fact that there is little clinical evidence that they help prevent coronary artery disease in the real world. These diets should be tested in clinical trials with a large enough patient group so that reasonable conclusions can be made about the results. Until that occurs, claims for low-fat diets remain simply that: unsubstantiated claims that may be misleading—and can cause harm to some people.

Think outside the Box

Let me interrupt your train of thought for a moment with a riddle. A man is on vacation with his son and is driving along a road when suddenly, he crashes into another car. The man dies, but the son is rushed to a nearby hospital. When the boy enters the operating room, however, the surgeon says, "I can't operate on him. He is my son!" How is this possible?

Many of us still picture all surgeons as being male. But in this case, the surgeon is the boy's mother. Medicine has been, and I suspect always will be, a gigantic riddle. A good physician is always thinking of innovative solutions to medical riddles such as heart disease that buck conventional wisdom. Yet the Fat Machine has become so powerful that it largely has pushed out other valid approaches to preventing coronary artery disease and heart attack.

Kilmer S. McCully, M.D., a researcher at Harvard Medical School behind the homocysteine story, which we will discuss in chapter 9, recalls how difficult it was for him to bring attention to the potential role of homocysteine, or "protein intoxication," and heart disease. The NIH was so consumed with the "cholesterol intoxication" story of coronary arteries that it virtually ignored other possibilities.

In the final analysis, the entire fat-cholesterol story is a reasonable one and should be respected. But it is also true that there is much more to heart disease that the quantity of fat in the diet and cholesterol levels. The message clearly is that there are other dietary ingredients that interact with dietary fats and that play major roles. In other words, there are other answers to the heart disease riddle. Take the following examples:

Saturated fat versus unsaturated fat. The French consume both saturated and unsaturated fat in substantial amounts. Yet their incidence of heart disease is much lower than in the United States. What is protecting French hearts? According to the Fat Machine, certain chemicals in red wine protect the French from heart disease. But, as we discuss in chapter 11, all alcohol is protective against heart attacks, not just red wine. And alcohol may play no role in this phenomenon at all. It may turn out to be some other dietary or genetic factor.

Total dietary fat. In the United States, the Fat Machine insists that less than 30 percent—and some say less than 20 percent—of total daily calories should come from fat in the diet. In Greece, approximately 40 percent of total daily calories come from fats, particularly in olive oil. Yet, the Greek rate of heart disease is substantially less than in the United States. The Italians, like the French and the Greeks, do not avoid eating meat or dairy products. In fact, they eat just about everything. However, the Italians usually don't eat in excess portions. Italians, Greeks, and French all have heart disease rates far below that of Americans.

This diet, popularly known as the Mediterranean Diet, was first promoted in the United States more than 30 years ago. Researchers at the University of Minnesota discovered that people who lived in any of seven Mediterranean countries had dramatically lower rates of coronary artery disease and heart attacks than Americans. In a 1999 study published in the journal *Circulation*, it was reported that the patients who followed the Mediterranean Diet, after having already had a heart attack, were 50 to 70 percent less likely than the comparison group to have another nonfatal or a fatal heart attack. In this study, conducted by Dr. Michel de Lorgeril and colleagues of Lyons, France, 30 percent of the calories in the Mediterranean Diet came from fat, compared with 34 percent from the control group. The Mediterranean group averaged 212 milligrams of cholesterol a day; the control group took in 312 milligrams. The Mediterranean group also ate more fiber, antioxidants, and B vitamins, all of which help slow the damage to the arteries that contributes to heart disease. Interestingly, after the study was ended, most of those on the Mediterranean Diet stayed on it.

In contrast, the Japanese diet contains fat levels that are extremely low. This is usually given as the explanation for their low rates of heart disease. This is reasonable, but Japanese cigarette smokers also seem impervious to coronary artery disease, unlike their American counterparts. As with the French, are other dietary factors involved? For example, could soy help protect Japanese smokers from coronary artery disease?

From these examples, it should be clear that there are many nutraceuticals that are as important, or even more important, than dietary fat intake and cholesterol levels in terms of your health. But because of the Fat Machine's overriding emphasis on fat and cholesterol, these other important factors have been pushed aside and ignored. The good news is that these factors finally have begun to be recognized and are entering the scene—through the back door.

Sensible Eating = Sensible Heart Protection

There are many other examples of diets that do seem to promote health and prolong life. But for any diet to work, you have to know who you are. The old adage, "Know thyself," is particularly appropriate here. We all need guidelines, but we need guidelines that are reasonable so that we can follow them.

I am not going to attempt to add "The DeFelice Diet" to the legion of diets that have come and gone, most of which have not helped people attain and maintain a desirable weight. It would be sheer folly to proclaim yet another diet. I do want to suggest, however, four general principles of a sound approach to eating that I believe will help the average person both eat and enjoy a heart-healthy diet. Balance is the foundation underlying these four simple suggestions. What I am recommending is doable for most people over the long term. This is where diets fail—people can't follow them for years or decades. But these guidelines take human nature into account, along with what we know about food and food ingredients and cardiovascular health today.

First, reach a "normal" weight and maintain that weight. Obesity is a serious problem and one that is difficult to solve. But exercise, a diet that matches up caloric intake and output, and eating less can all help you reach and maintain a desirable weight. It is very important to keep your weight steady.

Second, eat a mix of foods—plenty of vegetables, fruits, pasta, and fish. Learn to use olive oil. This will also help you keep your weight down. If you are obese, a diet high in vegetables will help you lose weight.

Third, take a reasonable approach to meat and dairy products.

These are high-energy foods and, I believe, have been mistakenly rejected by some experts because of their link to high cholesterol levels and obesity. How much you eat should be based on your weight. If you eat plenty of vegetables, fruits, and fish, then you can eat as much meat and as many dairy products as you want—as long as you maintain your normal weight. However, if you are already obese, it is wise to avoid the regular intake of meats (as well as other foods) until you have gotten your weight to a healthy level and are able to keep it there.

Fourth, the Cardiac Elixir completes the total cardiac approach. The Cardiac Elixir is particularly important to people who are obese and cannot lose weight, which results in increased cardiovascular risk.

Alcohol reduces your risk of heart disease by about 40 percent, raises "good" HDL cholesterol, and helps remove cholesterol from the body.

Vitamin E also reduces heart attack risk by about 40 percent and reduces "bad" LDL oxidation, that is, free radical activity as well.

Carnitine significantly reduces the risk of heart muscle damage due to ischemia or lack of oxygen to the heart usually caused by coronary artery disease.

Magnesium stops blood clotting, stabilizes heart function, and thus reduces the risk of heart muscle damage due to ischemia.

Vitamins B_6 and B_{12} and folic acid have been shown to reduce the risk of heart and coronary artery disease, and even more so when taken in combination.

Folic acid and alcohol in combination can reduced the risk of heart disease by 80 percent in women. The results of a similar study using folic acid and alcohol in men have not yet been released, but they are expected to confirm the results.

The clinical data now available indicate that the Cardiac Elixir will be good for your heart over the long run. I believe that the Cardiac Elixir is a very reasonable approach, based on good science and medicine, and one that the majority of people can easily follow.

Take a Helicopter to the Mountaintop

Though lessening, the resistance to the nutraceutical message remains quite strong. It is much easier, and more acceptable, for a leading medical or health authority to advocate a low-fat diet as an effective means of reducing the risk of heart disease than it is to recommend dietary supplementation. It takes courage for anyone to publicly state—with the same degree of confidence possessed by the proponents of low-fat diets—that it is important to take vitamin E to prevent heart attacks. Yet the clinical evidence supporting vitamin E supplementation is far greater than the evidence supporting the heart benefit claims concerning low-fat diets.

If I were asked what I would recommend to both patients at risk and healthy people—vitamin E or a low-fat diet to protect them against heart disease—I would recommend vitamin E. But I can assure you that most authorities would recommend the diet. They would make this recommendation in spite of the clinical data supporting the choice of vitamin E and despite the fact that people can't follow low-fat diets for one year, let alone a lifetime! I can assure you that it is easier to take one vitamin E pill a day than it is to follow a low-fat diet.

The question of how much and what kinds of fats should be in the diet is still a matter of controversy. There is evidence to support a wide range of approaches to healthy eating. I have outlined a simple plan, one that has the benefit of being easily implemented. To repeat, most recommended diets are too difficult for the average person to maintain over time.

Following a low-fat diet is like climbing to the top of a high mountain. Most experts recommend that people try to control their weight through a combination of diet and exercise, but we know that the average person finds it extremely difficult to do this. Most recommended diets are too difficult for the average person to maintain over time, and in general, obese people have an extraordinarily difficult time sticking to any low-fat eating regiment. It's also tough to stick with a program of regular exercise. We have to face the fact that most people just can't do it. They just don't make it to the mountaintop.

But taking the Cardiac Elixir is like flying to the mountaintop in a helicopter. The Cardiac Elixir provides a practical way for people who cannot manage their weight through diet and exercise to protect their hearts, and it offers those who are obese a potentially lifesaving solution. It seems to me that the Cardiac Elixir takes into account the complex mental and physical processes that are present in your body and their interaction with the complex human being who is living his or her life in this increasingly complex world. The Cardiac Elixir provides you with a doable way to decrease your reliance on the Fat Machine so that you can truly enhance and maintain your cardiac health.

CHAPTER FIVE

Heart Disease: The Natural Dimensions of Prevention

The circulatory system and its remarkable coordination of fluid dynamics, electrical impulses, and blood chemistries is one of the great wonders of nature. The heart, the potent pump at the center, which beats because, well, because it does, is enough to make a man downright reverent.

Yet, from a purely mechanistic point of view, the heart and our blood vessels strike me as pretty straightforward. The plain old plumbing metaphor comes to mind—just a pump and some pipes. Keep the pump well-oiled and in working order and the pipes clear and in good condition, and you won't have to call a cardiac surgeon. When it comes to taking care of your heart, the more down-to-earth idea should be your guiding principle. Maintenance of the plumbing is the key.

I don't mean to oversimplify. We're not simple machines, but organisms. And our cardiac pumps and pipes are part of a complex information feedback system, including electrical signals and messenger chemicals. Heart disease is most often multifactorial, brought on by a combination of causes. Though the genesis and details of each case of heart disease are unique, in broad brush, most of them have in common either a pump that's not at its best and/or some pipes that have been narrowed or damaged over time.

Your heart is a powerful muscle that pumps life-sustaining blood to every part of your body. It takes a lot to slow your heart down and even more to stop it. I'd like you to understand the different components of cardiac health and heart disease. If you understand the biology, you can make better decisions about what's best for you. Further, a knowledge of how heart disease develops will help you appreciate exactly how each of the nutraceuticals in the Cardiac Elixir can help keep you well.

You have to take care of three things: your heart, your blood vessels, and your blood. These three dimensions of prevention are, of course, interconnected. The condition of your vessels, for example, is greatly influenced by the chemistry of the blood that runs through them. But for purposes of clarity, to begin with, let's discuss them in isolation and explore the interrelations along the way.

Your Heart: The Engine of Life

You can think of your heart as two side-by-side pumps connected to one another. Each of the pumps has two chambers—an atrium on top, which receives the blood, and a ventricle below, which actually does the pumping.

The right side of your heart is responsible for what's called pulmonary circulation. It pumps your blood to your lungs, where two important things happen: (1) Your blood unloads carbon dioxide and (2) picks up oxygen. From there, the now oxygen-rich blood flows back to the left side of the heart. The left ventricle then pumps your blood—full of oxygen and other nutrients and able to pick up waste products—to every tissue in your body.

The Chambers of the Heart

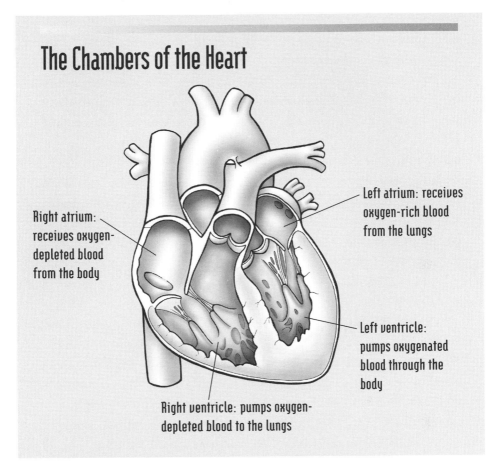

Right atrium: receives oxygen-depleted blood from the body

Left atrium: receives oxygen-rich blood from the lungs

Left ventricle: pumps oxygenated blood through the body

Right ventricle: pumps oxygen-depleted blood to the lungs

The left ventricle is the most powerful muscle in your heart. It has about 10 times as much muscle as the right ventricle. Why? The right ventricle only has to get your blood as far as your lungs, while the left ventricle has to fight gravity and squeeze blood all the way from your chest to the tiniest arteries in your brain. A healthy left ventricle is quite a device, about as forceful as a one-horsepower electric motor, stronger than many home appliances. The heart of an average person can pump about three quarts per minute.

In one respect, heart muscles are like any other. The more you use them, the stronger they stay. That's why exercise is such an important part of a cardiac health program. If your heart muscles don't get the work they need, they get weaker—just like your biceps or any other muscle in your body. If your heart muscles deteriorate, your heart can't pump as strongly.

Of course, your heart is critically different from muscles in one important respect. It's working all the time, not just when you're jogging or playing tennis. Your heart works even when you're just lying on the couch. So it's important that your heart's metabolism be operating at the highest level of efficiency.

Like any engine, the heart needs fuel to perform work. It prefers to use fats instead of carbohydrates because, gram for gram, fats produce considerably more energy. That's where carnitine comes in, since carnitine helps the heart and other muscles use fats as fuel. We'll see how in chapter 7.

Protecting the Passageways

Our vascular systems are amazing. It has been estimated that, counting even the most microscopic capillaries, an adult has almost 60,000 miles of blood vessels. Heading off problems with these vessels is crucial to cardiovascular health. The preventive trick is twofold: to keep the inside of the arteries clear and keep the arteries themselves as flexible, as elastic as possible. Here, too, the tasks are intertwined. If you keep the inside of the arteries clear, it's a good bet that they will stay resilient longer. But the bottom line is that the arteries must be both unobstructed and uncorroded.

In a perfectly healthy circulatory system, the vessels are clear passages for the flow of blood. Cardiac problems often start when cholesterol, calcium, or other substances start forming deposits on the inside of the arterial vessel walls. This is a disease called atherosclerosis.

What starts the initial formation of these deposits—called plaque or atheroma—is a matter of some debate. Some believe that plaque forms because of excess cholesterol in your blood. But plaque could also start forming as a result of a tiny injury in the vessel wall. Some researchers believe that these injuries are caused by bacterial infection or even the stress caused by bloodflow around a bend in a vessel.

The problem is that once the deposit starts to build, there's a continuing inflammatory reaction—a kind of cardiac snowball effect. Macrophages—white blood cells responsible for engulfing and ingesting bacteria and other microscopic invaders—are attracted to the spot, and they act like magnets for more cholesterol and other fats, adding to the biological buildup in the area. Plaques themselves get nourished by the same tiny blood vessels that feed the wall of the artery. The bigger one of these plaque deposits gets, the more these substances accumulate, narrowing the inside diameter of the vessel.

If the narrowing in one of more of the arteries feeding your heart gets severe enough, it can slow down the normal bloodflow to your heart. And if your heart isn't getting enough blood, it's

(continued on page 60)

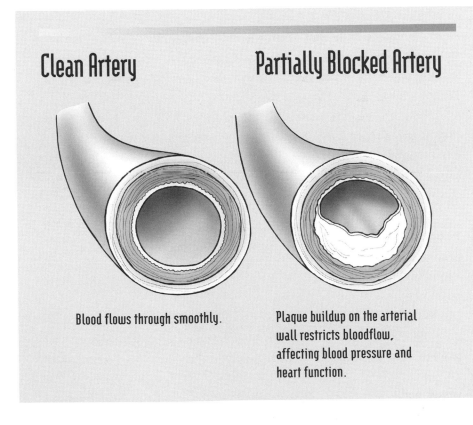

Clean Artery

Blood flows through smoothly.

Partially Blocked Artery

Plaque buildup on the arterial wall restricts bloodflow, affecting blood pressure and heart function.

Glossary of Heart Conditions

Throughout this book, I have used some technical terms that you might not be familiar with or that you might have trouble remembering as you read. To help you out, I've gathered many of these definitions in one place for quick and easy reference.

Atherosclerosis

What is it? A word frequently used interchangeably with arteriosclerosis (*sclerosis* means hardening), atherosclerosis is the thickening and hardening of the artery wall, initially through plaque buildup. Once the process begins, it is frequently accelerated by calcium deposits, hemorrhaging, and other pathological events. When atherosclerosis occurs in the vessels of heart muscle, it is called coronary artery atherosclerosis. Atherosclerosis can lead to ischemia, which can lead to heart cell damage, which can lead to a heart attack and to arrhythmia.

Signs and symptoms. Atherosclerosis is frequently symptom-free. Advanced coronary artery atherosclerosis can eventually result in angina pectoris, which does have symptoms, including pain that is similar to a heart attack but that often subsides with rest.

Coronary Artery Disease

What is it? Also known as *ischemic* heart disease or *myocardial ischemia*, coronary artery disease is an extremely common disorder and a leading cause of death. It is best defined as a narrowing of the coronary arteries and is usually caused by atherosclerosis. This narrowing restricts bloodflow to the heart, which in turn leads to damage or malfunction of the heart muscle.

Signs and symptoms. In its early stages, coronary artery disease can be symptomless, or "silent." Coronary artery disease can lead to angina pectoris, to heart attack, or to cardiomyopathy.

Myocardial Ischemia

What is it? Myocardial ischemia is a lack of blood and therefore oxygen to one or more arteries leading to the heart, usually the result of atherosclerosis of the affected artery. *Myocardial* refers to the heart, and *ischemia* means "not enough blood supply."

Signs and symptoms. There are two types: silent ischemia, which is symptom-free, and "noisy" ischemia, which is usually angina pectoris.

Angina Pectoris

What is it? Chest pain. Derived from two Latin words, *angina pectoris* literally means "pressure in the chest."

Signs and symptoms. People with angina pectoris experience pain similar to a heart attack. The pain usually begins in the center of the chest and can spread to the throat, upper jaw, back, shoulder blades, and arms. Other symptoms may include nausea, sweating, dizziness, and difficulty breathing. Unlike a heart attack, angina often subsides with rest.

Arrhythmia

What is it? Arrhythmia is an abnormality of the rhythm or rate of the heartbeat caused by a disturbance in the heart's electrical impulses. There are many different kinds of arrhythmia, both fatal and nonfatal. The most common form of fatal arrhythmia—and the most common cause of death following a heart attack—is called ventricular fibrillation. This affects the

(continued)

Glossary of Heart Conditions–Continued

beating action of the all-important left ventricle; as a result, the heart's pumping capacity becomes extremely inefficient, and oxygenated blood cannot reach the brain or even the heart muscle itself in sufficient quantities to maintain life. Arrhythmia can be associated with tachycardia, in which the heart beats faster than normal (more than 100 beats per minute), or with bradycardia, in which the heart beats slower than normal (fewer than 60 beats per minute).

Signs and symptoms. These include heart palpitations, dizziness, fainting, breathing difficulties, and chest pain.

Cardiomyopathy

What is it? Cardiomyopathy is a catchall term used to describe a heart that is too weak to pump blood efficiently. It is characterized by weakening of the left ventricle muscle—the part of the heart primarily responsible for pumping blood out to the body. This condition can eventually lead to congestive heart failure and is also closely associated with fatal arrhythmia.

Signs and symptoms. Fatigue, chest pain, palpitations, breathing difficulties, swelling of the legs and hands, and generalized weakness.

not getting the oxygen and other nutrients it needs. Then you have trouble: Coronary artery disease. Atherosclerosis. Plaque. Reduced bloodflow to the heart is also often called ischemic heart disease or myocardial ischemia. If your heart isn't getting enough blood, it's not getting the oxygen and other nutrients that it needs.

If the blockage is severe enough, you'll feel the problem yourself through a chest pain called angina pectoris. People who experience this generally have a sensation of pressure, tightening, or burning. The pain usually starts in the chest, but it often radiates into the left arm and left shoulder and sometimes into the back or even up into the jaw.

Hypertension

What is it? Abnormally and chronically high blood pressure. Hypertension increases your risk of developing heart failure, stroke, and coronary artery disease.

Signs and symptoms. Hypertension often has no symptoms and goes undetected until a routine physical exam. In severe cases, hypertension can cause shortness of breath, headaches, visual problems, and giddiness.

Myocardial Infarction

What is it? A heart attack. It is the result of a significant loss of blood supply to the heart, which leads to the death of cells in one or more parts of the muscle.

Signs and symptoms. Heart attack pain is similar to angina, except that it persists for 30 minutes or more and is not relieved by rest. The characteristic symptom is a sudden pain in the center of the chest. The pain can also radiate into the throat, upper jaw, back, shoulder blades, and left arm. Other symptoms may include restlessness; nausea; sweating; dizziness; difficulty breathing; and cold, clammy skin.

Patients whose coronary arteries are partially blocked most often have pain during or after exertion. The heart tries to speed up and generate extra pressure to send more blood to the hardworking muscles, both in the heart itself and throughout the body. But since the coronary arteries are greatly narrowed, the heart can't get the blood where it's needed, and pain comes with the effort. The discomfort usually stops shortly after exertion stops.

Sometimes, angina pain can be brought on by emotional stress, anger, or fear, all of which make the heart start beating faster, increasing the workload. Though the reasons aren't clear, angina can also be triggered by eating meals and by extreme cold or heat, probably because the heart has to work harder to supply blood to the liver and intestines in order to sustain the process of digestion.

But here's the crucial fact about angina: By the time you have any symptoms at all, you could be well on your way to heart disease. Generally, a coronary vessel has to be 50 percent obstructed before you feel chest pain. Some people have even greater blockages without the warning of angina pain. Unbeknownst to you, the blood vessels in your heart could be gradually but steadily narrowing. It's difficult to estimate how many people have so-called silent ischemia, but there's no doubt that the numbers are very high and that many of the apparently healthy people who are suddenly stricken by heart attacks were carrying the time bomb of ischemia in their arteries.

This is a common situation in which carnitine can offer vital cardio-protection. I explain it in more detail in chapter 7. But for now, understand that high levels of carnitine can help your heart get the energy that it needs even if the flow of blood is compromised by a blockage.

Keeping the Arteries Young

Preserving the diameter of the arteries is just job one when it comes to vascular health. We also need to take care of the arteries themselves. The healthiest arteries are flexible and resilient, able to dilate and contract quickly and easily when your body requires more bloodflow. To understand the importance of elasticity in your arteries, consider what happens during one of those adrenaline moments of excitement or fear.

Let's say you see a car coming at you. Your eyes send the danger message to your brain. Your brain instantly instructs your adrenal glands, located on top of your kidneys, to produce more adrenaline, also known as epinephrine. Why? Adrenaline does three things. First, it makes the blood vessels in your intestines constrict. Second, it makes your heart beat faster, greatly increasing the amount of blood that it can pump. Third, it dilates the vessels to your muscles as well as the vessels to your heart. The result? More blood is pumped to your legs so that you can run out of the way of the onrushing car. Healthy arteries can constrict or dilate like this with no problem. But if your blood vessels are not in good shape—if they've been hardened by plaque buildup inside them—they just don't contract as quickly and easily as they need to, nor do they dilate as quickly as they need to in other situations.

If your arteries are clogged with plaque, an adrenal moment is a kind of mini trauma. Sometimes, this kind of trauma can make a clot, called a thrombosis, form on top of the plaque inside a coronary vessel. The result can be a complete blockage of the vessel, which kills cells in the heart. The common term for this condition is heart attack. Lots of people have heart attacks when their adrenal glands are stimulated—right after they've been angry, frightened, or sexually excited.

But plaque buildup inside arteries is just one reason why the walls of the arteries become more rigid. They also can be damaged over time by high blood pressure. The constant mechanical stress on the artery walls can diminish their flexibility, just as constantly pulling a rubber band can make it lose its snap. At the same time, constant stress on the walls may cause microscopic injuries around which plaques develop. Science has attributed plaque buildup to genetic factors, which influence the structure and function of the interior linings of blood vessels.

Emotional stress can also compromise blood vessels. There is some evidence that hot-tempered people or people under stress are at greater risk of heart disease than the serene among us. The repeated constriction of the arteries caused by many angry moments is debilitating to the vessel walls.

Independent of blood pressure or personality issues, arteries just tend to get a little less resilient as time goes by. If that explanation sounds woefully unscientific, I plead guilty on behalf of medical science. Though we have some tantalizing leads, we still don't yet fully understand the process of aging.

We do, however, have one model of aging that explains a lot—

the oxidation model. It goes like this: Our bodies age as a result of the molecules called free radicals. These are unstable oxygen molecules that are lacking an electron and roam your bloodstream looking for the electron they're missing. They steal electrons from other molecules in a damaging process called oxidation. It's often pointed out that oxidation is the process that makes metal rust and makes a banana turn brown. Free radical damage is believed to be responsible for cellular damage, which is at the heart of the aging process.

This is where nutraceuticals offer hope. Many of them—including vitamin E, a Cardiac Elixir ingredient—are antioxidants. By offering up their own electrons to the rampaging free radicals, they can limit the damage done by free radicals. There is strong evidence that vitamin E can slow down the aging of arteries and help keep them more resilient and better able to cope with the demands of vasodilation and constriction.

Your Blood: The River of Life

In *The Royal Family*, a play by George Kaufman, one of the characters walks in on a family argument and offers a witticism that applies to heart health. "I see blood is thicker than usual," he observes, twisting the old blood-is-thicker-than-water loyalty cliché.

To keep your heart healthy, it's important to keep your blood chemistry in balance. The consistency of your blood has to be just right. Too thin, and it won't clot properly. Too thick, and it won't flow smoothly. The viscosity of your blood is by no means the only important issue when it comes to blood chemistry. To cite our plumbing metaphor, if the water running through the pipes in your home is loaded with impurities, sediments will gradually build up inside the pipes, reducing the flow through the system. Optimal heart health requires blood chemistry that is fine-tuned in respect to several different factors.

Cholesterol. No doubt you know about the importance of con-

Saving the Fringe Areas in Heart Attacks

The medical community used to believe that all of the heart muscle that's supposed to be fed by a blocked coronary artery was doomed to death by oxygen starvation within 20 to 30 minutes. They believed that the demise of these cells was inevitable, and that a process called apoptosis (programmed cell death) automatically takes over when the cells are near death. Once your body detects that cells are wounded, it sends in hormones and messenger substances that program these cells to die.

Researchers have discovered, however, that cell death may not be inevitable for every oxygen-starved heart cell. There is a fringe area where the heart muscle may not die immediately. Some of the muscle cells in this fringe area may remain in a kind of suspended animation. Despite oxygen-deprivation during an ischemic event, these heart cells may be capable of surviving or even regenerating. This means that doctors may soon concentrate their efforts on keeping as much of this fringe area alive as possible. To this end, researchers are actively working on agents that could counteract the process of cell death in ischemic heart tissue.

There is strong evidence that carnitine, the centerpiece of the Cardiac Elixir, may be able to buy time for those heart cells in the fringe area. If enough heart cells stay alive in one or more of these fringe areas, programmed cell death may not occur, and the heart muscle might survive.

trolling the level of cholesterol in your blood. But to appreciate how cardiovascular nutraceuticals can protect you, it's important to understand that cholesterol actually changes the structure and function of arteries. That's why high levels of cholesterol can put you at higher risk.

Cholesterol could use a public relations agent, since it has such a bad reputation. Some of this fatlike substance is vital to our well-being. When you eat it, it's synthesized in your liver and plays a central role in many metabolic processes, including the manufacture of hormones, especially sex hormones and adrenal gland hormones. Cholesterol is also an essential component of cell membranes and the bile acids, which we need for proper digestion. Our bodies need cholesterol. Our blood carries it to every cell.

But here's an important wrinkle. Cholesterol, a fat, isn't water-soluble, meaning that it can't dissolve in our blood. So it travels around as a particle, encased in a special type of blood-soluble protein called a lipoprotein. Lipoproteins come in two varieties: high-density lipoproteins (HDLs) and low-density lipoproteins (LDLs).

The HDLs are commonly called good cholesterol. They actually benefit your heart by acting like little janitors, removing cholesterol from your tissues and arteries and transporting it to HDL receptors in your liver, which store it safely for future use.

The LDLs, or bad cholesterol, are the heart threat. Here's the pathology sequence. If you have too much of this kind of lipoprotein in your blood, the LDL molecules combine with excess oxygen in your circulatory system. This LDL-oxygen marriage attracts the attention of your macrophages (white blood cells) that react to this combined molecule as an invader. The macrophages pick up the oxidized LDL and convert it to foam cells—one of the integral components of plaque.

Homocysteine. Many persuasive studies indicate that high levels of an amino acid called homocysteine are associated with heart disease. Homocysteine is a by-product of your body's protein synthesis. Normally, it's recycled over and over again as protein. But when you have more than you need, it appears that homocysteine may contribute to buildup of the substances in plaque. We don't yet know precisely how or why this happens, but clinical trials are under way to explore the link between lower homocysteine levels and a reduced incidence of coronary artery disease.

Clotting factors. You've probably heard about taking aspirin to prevent ischemia or heart attack. Many doctors recommend it because the active ingredient in aspirin—acetylsalicylic acid—works to thwart the aggregation of platelets and so the formation of plaques. If our blood doesn't have the right amounts of any of the substances—including the proteins thrombin and fibrinogen, which control the complex clotting process—we're at higher cardiac risk.

There are basically five ways to control the chemistry of your blood: (1) by what you eat, (2) by exercise, (3) by your thoughts, (4) with drugs, or (5) with nutraceutical supplements. Later, when we explore the ingredients of the Cardiac Elixir, you'll learn how nutraceuticals can play a pivotal part in balancing your blood chemistries.

High Blood Pressure and High Risk

Blood pressure, the force with which your blood flows through your arteries, is a key heart-health factor that is influenced by all three dimensions of heart disease prevention. If your heart itself isn't working at top efficiency, your blood pressure can be too low to get blood and nutrients to all parts of your body. If your vessel walls are hardened, they can't dilate and constrict when they need to in response to hormonal surge. This can contribute to high blood pressure.

Even if your heart is working well and your arteries are in good shape, you can have blood pressure problems. Your blood pressure is controlled by hormones produced by your kidneys and your adrenal gland as well as by substances produced by the arteries themselves. Nutraceuticals can help with blood pressure problems in a variety of ways. For example, angiotensin II, one of the key hormones, responds to magnesium, an important ingredient in the Cardiac Elixir.

People with high blood pressure are at higher risk for atherosclerosis, heart attack, and heart disease caused by oxygen deprivation to the cardiac tissues. As we'll see, nutraceuticals can help.

Diabetes and Heart Disease

People with diabetes are at especially high risk of heart disease. Indeed, the incidence of heart disease among people with diabetes is 8 to 10 times greater than in the general population. Most people don't equate diabetes with heart disease, but insulin plays an important role in both the growth and repair of cells throughout our bodies. Since blood vessels are living organisms requiring constant growth and repair, maintaining a healthy circulatory system is a constant challenge for those with diabetes.

Diabetes also comes with other traits that work against heart health, including an increased sensitivity to angiotensin II, the hormone that makes blood vessels constrict, and a tendency toward platelet aggregation, or clotting. These factors often add up to not enough blood and, therefore, not enough oxygen, getting to the heart and other vital organs.

Many people with diabetes, especially those with type 2 (adult onset, or non-insulin-dependent) diabetes, are magnesium-deficient. As we will see in chapter 10, supplements of this nutraceutical can help reduce the severity of these risk factors.

Heart Attacks and Beyond

Heart attacks happen when a blockage of the coronary artery is so severe that it cuts off the blood supply to one or more areas of your heart. Heart attacks, also called myocardial infarctions, are usually caused either by the plaque buildup of advanced coronary artery disease, thrombosis (a blood clot), or an intense spasm that obstructs one or more arteries with plaque or a clot. The tissues of the heart that can't get oxygen-carrying blood start to die.

Though many people think of a heart attack as a sudden, usually fatal episode, that's not an accurate picture. The seriousness of an infarction depends on how big an area of the heart is damaged and which area. Some heart attacks can be painless and even relatively harmless. On the other hand, if the so-called pacemaker cells, which produce the electrical currents that stimulate your heartbeat, are affected, you can have a cardiac rhythm disorder, or arrhythmia, which can lead to ventricular fibrillation, the most severe type of arrhythmia, and lethal cardiac arrest.

If a heart attack damages a large part of your heart, you may develop cardiomyopathy, a catchall term for a heart that's too weak to work efficiently as a pump. Sometimes, in the early stages of cardiomyopathy, your uninjured heart muscle can stretch to compensate for the lost pumping action of the damaged muscle. But often, cardiomyopathy can lead to congestive heart failure. The weakened left ventricle can't pump blood throughout the body, and the blood starts backing up into the lungs. Then the serious symptoms of heart failure set in—shortness of breath, fluid buildup in your lungs and legs, dangerously low blood pressure, and/or overall weakness.

Medicine and Certainty

I've covered a lot of ground in this chapter, and even so, I've only given a cursory sense of how cardiovascular disease develops. What's more, new developments in heart disease are continually emerging. For example, there is some preliminary research evidence to suggest that heart disease, and especially heart attacks, may be caused by infection or inflammation within our arteries. But any conclusive judgments about this possibility are a way off. Even if this theory is borne out, it won't diminish the importance of keeping arteries healthy and clear but merely add to our understanding of exactly how they get compromised.

Medicine is an imprecise art and science. And heart disease is especially vexing because it sometimes seems capricious. We've all heard the stories of the overweight smoker who exercises by lifting pastrami sandwiches and lives, in fine fettle, until he's 94. Conversely, we've all heard stories of the marathoning, supplement-taking vegetarian who is stricken by heart disease at an early age. But remember this: The reason why you hear these stories is because they're news. Don't let one particular tale of either dissolute longevity or unrewarded virtue become an excuse to be careless about your heart health.

To be sure, there is chaos afoot. We still don't understand all the reasons why people have heart attacks. But cardiac care is all about doing everything you can to increase your chances of staying well.

There is no such thing as a small health edge. Each of the nutraceuticals in the Cardiac Elixir works against one or more of the pathological processes that contribute to heart disease. Here are some of the ways in which that happens.

■ *Carnitine and magnesium help nourish and regulate your heart.*

■ *Vitamin E protects your blood vessels.*

■ *The B vitamins and alcohol control your blood chemistry.*

Taken together, these discrete health advantages amount to a powerful shield, a recipe of nature's medicines that can greatly increase your chances of staying well.

PART TWO

The Cardiac Elixir

CHAPTER SIX

Why an Elixir?

One of my favorite operas, Gaetano Donizetti's *L'Elisir d'Amore* (*Elixir of Love*), deals with the subject of nutraceuticals. In it, Nemorino, a none-too-attractive peasant, attempts to win the heart of the popular and seemingly unattainable Adina. His efforts, thwarted by his shyness, appear destined to comic opera failure. But then he meets the flamboyant Dr. Dulcamara, who offers Nemorino a mysterious love potion comprised of wine and many other ingredients. Nemorino swallows the elixir and is suddenly imbued with new confidence that he can successfully woo the object of his affection. By the time the final curtain drops, Dr. Dulcamara's cardiac love mixture has successfully turned Adina's head. She has fallen madly in love with the self-effacing Italian. Nemorino and Adina live happily ever after, thanks to the very first successful Cardiac Elixir on record.

You may be asking yourself, "What does this so-called love mixture have to do with a Cardiac Elixir?" Precisely this: Nemorino believed that the elixir was a mixture of magical ingredients and that its strength was not in its individual components, but in all of the ingredients interacting and working together.

What's in a Name?

Throughout this book, I support my views of the effectiveness of nutraceuticals with conclusions published in respectable medical journals, as well as my own personal judgment and the opinions of my colleagues. That's because I want to make a convincing case, and physicians are trained to recommend only drugs that have been shown to be effective based on clinical studies that have been published in acceptable medical journals.

It's not easy for a clinical study to get published in a respected medical journal. The manuscript is first reviewed by medical experts, whose identity is kept secret. They critique the study's methods, procedures, and conclusions. Not infrequently, they tear it apart. Generally speaking, the more prestigious the journal, the higher the caliber of the reviewers and the more rigorous their requirements.

These detailed comments and queries are then sent back to the clinical researchers, who must respond satisfactorily to the reviewers' criticisms and questions. If the study is poorly designed or comes to questionable conclusions, it will usually be rejected.

Some of the journals with the most credibility among the medical profession include the *Journal of the American Medical Association* (*JAMA*), the *New England Journal of Medicine*, the *Archives of Internal Medicine*, the *Annals of Medicine*, *Circulation*, the *American Journal of Cardiology*, and *The Lancet*. There are others.

A study published in a lesser journal may also have value. But the better the journal, the higher the probability that doctors will consider its findings believable.

Taking one of the nutraceuticals in the Cardiac Elixir simply isn't enough. You need to take every one of them. Why? Because all nutraceuticals don't work for everyone. And because the causes of heart disease are so varied. The Cardiac Elixir gives you much broader cardiovascular insurance than any single nutraceutical.

Why Nutraceuticals Don't Work for Everyone

You cannot be sure that you are the particular person who will benefit from a specific nutraceutical, because vitamin E, alcohol, folic acid, and other components of the Cardiac Elixir only work in a certain percentage of people.

Take vitamin E, for instance. In clinical studies, this vitamin has been found to reduce cardiovascular events such as heart attacks by about 40 percent. But what about the other 60 percent? Should we forget about them? Of course not.

Also, over time, even vitamin E alone will not be enough to protect all of the fortunate people in the 40 percent group. The truth is, over time, many of those who take vitamin E will eventually experience heart attacks anyway. Again, should we forget about them? And again, I say no. It goes against the good practice of medicine.

Additionally, it is difficult for you to know if a particular nutraceutical is working for you as an individual. The beauty of the Cardiac Elixir is that if one or two of the ingredients in the Elixir don't work for you because of your unique biological composition, you can be fairly certain that one or more of the other components will.

Furthermore, when it comes to nutraceuticals, one plus one can equal 10. Nutraceuticals often work together. Alcohol alone, for instance, may reduce the risk of heart disease in women by 40 percent. But as has been reported in the *Journal of the American Medical Association*, women who take alcohol plus folic acid had about an 80 percent reduction in cardiac risk. Likewise, carnitine generates adenosine triphosphate (ATP), the energy molecule your heart needs. That's good for your heart, but you can protect it even more if you're taking magnesium, which stabilizes the ATP molecule. The two substances add up to more, in terms of results, than either of them separately.

The more nutraceutical ingredients you take, the broader the medical promise.

Different Nutraceuticals Treat
Different Aspects of Heart Disease

You need a number of substances for maximum protection because heart disease, like all diseases, involves many different pathological processes. The more of these pathological processes you can attack, the better your odds of staving off disease. It's only logical to prevent or fight the multiple processes of impending disease with a multipronged, rationally designed mixture: the Cardiac Elixir.

Let's start with your circulatory system. Fatty plaque buildup in the inner lining of your arteries, also known as atherosclerosis, can be caused by many different factors in the blood: the buildup of free oxygen radicals; excess homocysteine; blood clots, which form blockages; and/or the accumulation of cholesterol.

Different nutraceuticals are effective against each of these processes. Vitamin E can help you fight off the free oxygen radical activities, and the B vitamins can help keep your homocysteine levels down. At the same time, alcohol (in moderation), can not only slow down the clot formation process but also raise your "good" high-density lipoprotein (HDL) cholesterol level, all of which reduces your risk of atherosclerosis.

But what if you're a person who, knowingly or unknowingly, already has lots of plaque buildup? Taking vitamin E, the B vitamins, and so on might help you prevent more plaque buildup. So I still strongly recommend them.

But they won't necessarily protect your heart itself. The atherosclerosis already in your blood vessels may make you prone to ischemia, also known as lack of oxygen to your heart—and that makes you more prone to heart cell damage and heart attacks. Furthermore, if you've already had a bout of angina pectoris or had a heart attack, many of the same processes that may have led to your first bout of these ailments are ongoing and could lead to subsequent episodes, perhaps even to a fatal heart attack.

Carnitine, another critical ingredient in the Cardiac Elixir, can protect your heart against these prospects with its ability to generate ATP, or cellular energy. Taking carnitine could prevent a heart attack or prevent your heart's cells from dying in the course of a heart attack. At the same time, magnesium stabilizes the ATP-production process, helping to optimize the heart energy system. Likewise, continuing to take vitamin E is important as well for people who have had a heart attack because it will continue to keep treating the disease process that led to the first heart attack and, hopefully, will prevent the next one.

The evidence that the core ingredients of the Cardiac Elixir work together as a team is compelling. I could go on and on about the many virtues of these interactions. But it comes down to this concept: Since heart disease involves multiple abnormal processes, and since we have not yet discovered a single cure for all its causes and manifestations, it makes powerful medical sense to give combinations of nutraceuticals in an attempt to diminish its potential for devastating physical and mental impact.

Multiple causes of disease call for multiple treatments of these causes. That's what you get with the Cardiac Elixir.

Getting the Message Out:
A Double-Edged Sword

As you know, I've been labeled "the Don Quixote of Nutraceuticals" because I've been tilting at the windmills of conventional medical opinion for a few decades now (and for most of that time, nobody was listening). I tried to educate the public and my professional colleagues about the importance of combining nutraceuticals, and my message fell upon deaf ears.

Fortunately, times have changed.

Everybody used to be enthralled with artificial molecules. They were right. Can you imagine a life without pharmaceuticals? Many of us would have long succumbed to the ravages of heart disease, cancer, arthritis, diabetes, or another fatal ailment.

But progress in medicine has always meant proving the experts

Clinical Realities

What makes a study acceptable to reputable physicians and scientists? First and foremost, it must be well-controlled, or at least reasonably well-controlled. Some of the main types of well-controlled studies that medical professionals accept include:

The "double-blind, placebo-controlled" clinical study. This is the gold standard—the most unbiased and convincing type of study possible, according to most physicians. Placebo-controlled means that some patients will get the substance to be evaluated, while others will receive a placebo: an inert substance, like a sugar pill. The reason for the placebo control group is that many people seem to get better just by thinking they're on medication. Placebo alone can improve the signs and symptoms of up to half the patients suffering from such diseases as depression, pain, hypertension, and arthritis. Only by comparing the placebo group to the substance under study can researchers make a true comparison. Double-blind means that neither the patient nor the physician/researcher knows what is in the pill or product under study or even who is receiving what substance. Bottom line: Such studies can objectively demonstrate that only people who take the substance under study will show an effect, while those who do not take the substance will show little or no effect.

wrong. There was a great need to expand the boundaries of medical treatment beyond pharmaceuticals, to include nutraceuticals. I have been convinced for a long time that the Cardiac Elixir can be an integral component of total medical care—and a great leap forward in cardiovascular health.

That's why in 1976, alarmed by the lack of discovery and availability of natural substances that treat or prevent illness, I formed the Foundation for Innovation in Medicine, or FIM. A nonprofit educational organization based in New Jersey and New York, FIM closely monitors worldwide activities in medical research and supports and encourages American clinical research, particularly in the area of nutraceuticals and other natural substances. It also actively

Epidemiological studies. These analyze large populations. The Harvard studies of physicians and nurses that you'll read about in this book are a good example of carefully controlled epidemiological studies. They analyze the diet of comparable groups over long periods of time and find persuasive differences between the incidence of heart disease over time among people with low vitamin E intake compared to those with high vitamin E intake.

Multicenter studies. As the name suggests, multi-center studies are those conducted in more than one place. They are necessary when researchers have to go to several centers to find suitable candidates in sufficient numbers for their studies. If you want to show that a substance reduces the incidence of heart attacks by 10%, for instance, you may need to study thousands of patients to show a statistically convincing effect.

Meta-analysis. This is a method of evaluating several or many studies that have already been conducted. Each of these studies may not be powerful enough to be convincing on its own, but the pooled evidence could be compelling. Gingko biloba achieved recognition for helping cognitive function, for instance, based on a meta-analysis of 12 European studies. The separate studies showed a positive effect that was questionable, but the cumulative results, which were all in the same direction, were more convincing.

educates the government on the need to enact new laws that encourage medical discovery. Its conferences, which I host in New York or Washington twice a year, are a forum for sharing the latest information about the science, medicine, and politics of nutraceuticals with the international community—medical doctors, industry pharmaceutical specialists, patients, and healthy people. For many years, these conferences were a fringe phenomenon.

Then, in 1983, the public embraced its first bona fide message of nutraceutical hope. The popularization of calcium by the mass media to prevent postmenopausal osteoporosis was the beginning of the Nutraceutical Revolution. And possibly because of calcium, today, I'm no Don Quixote. The critics have been silenced with solid, impressive clinical evidence. The public and my colleagues are finally ready to hear and accept the nutraceutical message.

I have been fortunate to witness the Nutraceutical Revolution and the growing desire of Americans to tap into the powers of natural substances to enhance their health. Today, more than 100 million people in the United States are taking nutraceuticals every day, and I would venture to say that a substantial portion of their intake includes cardiovascular nutraceuticals. More and more physicians now accept nutraceutical mixtures or elixirs as an approach to prevent and treat heart disease. In fact, it is estimated that 8 out of every 10 physicians are taking vitamin E, and many of those doctors are recommending this supplement to their patients. Some are also beginning to take—and recommend—folic acid, vitamin B_{12}, and vitamin B_6. Modest consumption of alcohol is becoming standard advice that doctors not only cautiously endorse, but practice themselves.

Spreading the Word about Nutraceuticals

I am delighted that the American public is finally ready to listen to the fact that nutraceuticals have a major impact on reducing heart disease and even heart attacks, both fatal and nonfatal.

I am very gratified that more and more people are going to their doctors and asking, "What about vitamin E?" or "Will coenzyme Q_{10} help my arteries?" They want every opportunity to protect their bodies against disease. They sense that Mother Nature knows best. But their enthusiasm raises a serious dilemma.

Jane Henney, M.D., the commissioner of the FDA, has stated that about 50 percent of the adult population in the United States is taking dietary supplement nutraceuticals daily, often consuming multiple tablets or capsules. Some people are taking vitamin E, others are taking the B vitamins. Some are taking both, along with a handful of whatever supplement of the week is featured on CNN.

Most are not making their decisions—or determining their doses—based on a clear rationale or on good science. There's a world of nutraceutical chaos out there.

We have an impressive body of evidence clearly demonstrating that a core group of natural substances known as nutraceuticals can play an important role in the prevention and treatment of heart disease and the proper functioning of blood vessels.

We know that a specific mixture of these substances is the most effective way to maintain cardiac health.

We have compelling data telling us that your heart needs carnitine to protect itself against an episode of oxygen deprivation. People with diabetes need magnesium supplementation to protect their hearts and blood vessels. Everyone needs vitamin E to lower their risk of developing fat deposits in their arteries. Moderate drinking can prevent heart disease.

These are facts. The clinical research bears them out.

But which substances should you take? What's the right combination? How much should you take? Nobody knows.

It is clearly time to educate both health care professionals and the public about which nutraceuticals can normalize many disease conditions that ultimately affect the heart.

This book is the first attempt that I'm aware of to provide the American public and physicians with the latest findings about effective cardiovascular nutraceuticals. It is also the first time that all these ingredients have been prescribed in one place. And it's the only resource you'll find that's entirely based on good clinical evidence.

When I talk about good clinical evidence, I'm talking about expert physicians evaluating published studies, coming to an agreement or consensus about its potential for medical use, and then communicating their findings to the mass media. I'm talking about objective analysis of the latest facts available to medical science today. Certainly, that's been my focus as a clinician and as a physician.

Every recommendation in this book is driven primarily by clinical data derived from studies on human subjects and published in respected medical and scientific journals. The analysis of this information, supported by many other respected physician colleagues, is available in no other published material to date.

(continued on page 84)

How to Make the Most of Nutraceuticals

There are three main ways that you can make the most of nutraceuticals to benefit your health, whether for your overall well-being or to prevent or treat specific conditions, such as heart disease, cancer, or fatigue.

1. Be aware of the importance of clinical data and research. The only way to cut the enormous cost of illness to our society is to reduce disease. And how do you reduce disease? One good way is to educate yourself about the substances that can prevent and/or treat disease. Stay hungry for medical proof. Continue enlightening yourself about the good clinical research that's out there about natural substances that can fortify you against disease. Read about the benefits of fish oil, fiber, vitamin C, beta-carotene, vitamin E, *Ginkgo biloba*, folic acid, *Echinacea*, St. John's wort, cranberry juice, and other such substances. Talk them over with your physician and take those substances that medical experts recommend, based on published clinical studies. The public's appetite for nutraceutical knowledge will feed the demand for more clinical research into these substances.

2. Be aware that, in general, there is no single nutraceutical "magic bullet." Up until now, the medical and scientific communities have been conditioned to seek, and then administer, a "magic bullet"—one substance or approach that will relieve people of their ills, or at least their symptoms—and provide continuing good health. This philosophy is hopelessly out of touch with medical reality. As a total approach, it has created numerous failures, followed by inevitable disappointment and suspicion. It's bad medicine, plain and simple. This book is about good medicine.

Your heart responds to a mixture of ingredients that maintain its integrity. Just as a good meal turns on all bodily systems to keep the mind and the body going, just as each and every natural hormone can perform a variety of healing functions in your body, the right combination of nutraceuticals can enhance your heart health.

3. Work closely with your physician. Although classically trained physicians tend to rely on drugs and surgery to treat hearts that are already ill, many are rapidly becoming positively disposed toward other forms of therapy—particularly preventive measures considered "alternative" in nature.

Don't join the 40 to 50 percent of Americans who take supplements and opt to not tell their doctors—either because they don't trust their doctor's counsel on these supplements or because they don't want to go against their physicians if supplements are not prescribed. You and your doctor can be a powerful and effective working team. But you must first respect each other and trust each other enough to share information about therapy and supplementation.

This advice is particularly important if you're already taking pharmaceutical medication. Right now, some of you may be taking statins to lower your cholesterol or anti-arrhythmia medication to keep your heartbeat regular. If you suffer from angina, you may be on nitroglycerines, calcium channel blockers, or beta blockers. You may also need drugs to retard clotting of your blood (anti-platelet drugs, anticoagulants, or "blood-thinners"). It's essential that you continue taking these medications under the direction of your doctor. And it's just as important that you share your nutraceutical intake with your doctor. Although the individual chapters of the book will point out the potential benefits or harmful side effects of the nutraceutical-drug interaction, the truth is that there are few data on this very important phenomenon.

I can see some of you shaking your heads in disbelief, and thinking, "My physician doesn't know anything about cardiovascular nutraceuticals. Why bother aggravating the doctor with information that is just going to make him or her mad at me?"

Don't underestimate him or her: More and more physicians are becoming comfortable with these substances. Although your doctor will probably only approve of nutraceuticals that are backed up with clinical support, he or she is seeing such support more and more. And we're at a point in the information explosion where you're going to have to make your decisions based on a dialogue with your caregiver. You will have to develop an entirely different connection with your physician in order to ensure that you are taking nutraceuticals that are safe and effective for your particular situation.

Hand your doctor this book, which has the latest information available. Why not start the dialogue right now?

This is not some kind of fad cure-all. The Cardiac Elixir that I propose is supported by the results of clinical research from around the world. Each of the ingredients in the Elixir has been researched in multiple clinical trials by trained researchers and highly respected physicians. Each has withstood rigorous scientific examination.

My Response to My Critics

Some of my colleagues in academic medicine would object to this prescription. They are what I call purists. They would ask me how many people have been taking this Elixir successfully. I would have to say one: me. I've been using carnitine for 25 years, and over the past few years, I have added the rest of my Cardiac Elixir to my intake.

They would then demand costly long-term and ironclad studies, featuring all the ingredients in the Elixir. Before they would recommend it for the prevention and treatment of heart disease, they would want to determine conclusively that this exact combination is safe and effective. While this course of action might be prudent for a new pharmaceutical, I would strongly resist any effort that would delay the use of the Cardiac Elixir.

To those of my colleagues who want to wait until all these gold-standard studies are complete, I say this:

It is improbable that these studies will be completed and published within the near or even the distant future. The costs to companies would be far too high. And the current clinical data regarding the components of the Elixir are persuasive well within the bounds of medical acceptability. In fact, clinical studies on many cholesterol-lowering drugs—to use just one example—have been shown, in very sophisticated clinical trials, to report similar cardiac protective effects to those of certain nutraceuticals. That is why so many doctors are now taking and recommending cardiovascular nutraceuticals, such as alcohol, folic acid, and vitamin E.

Likewise, my skeptical colleagues, when your patient has myocardial ischemia, heart failure, cardiac arrhythmias, arthritis, fatigue, and constipation, you are likely to prescribe combinations of drugs to treat these conditions. In practically all such cases, these exact combinations have never been evaluated in any clinical studies. Why are you raising the bar on nutraceuticals alone?

I believe that many lives would unnecessarily be lost due to heart attacks during the many years that it would take to complete these studies. In addition, the available information indicates that safety of these nutraceuticals is presently not a major problem. The benefits of taking the Elixir seem to far outweigh the risks.

There is no need to conduct double-blind studies for each ingredient or search for a potential magic bullet in the combination, as my academic colleagues and the federal government would prefer.

Simply put, we have a clear choice: Take the Cardiac Elixir or not. Many physicians and I have no doubts about our verdict. We are taking them.

Here's my personal recommendation for the Cardiac Elixir.

Note: If you are on any medication, be sure to check with your physician.

Carnitine	1,500 to 3,000 milligrams daily, divided into two doses, 12 hours apart
Vitamin E	400 international units daily
Folic acid	400 micrograms daily
Vitamin B$_6$	400 to 500 milligrams daily
Vitamin B$_{12}$	500 to 1,000 micrograms daily
Magnesium	400 to 500 milligrams daily, divided into two doses, 12 hours apart
*Chromium**	500 to 1,000 micrograms
*Alcohol***	One drink daily for women, one to two drinks for men. A drink is a 12-ounce bottle of beer or wine cooler, 4- to 5-ounce glass of wine, or 1.25 to 1.5 ounces of 80-proof distilled spirits.

*Chromium supplementation is only recommended for people with diabetes.
**Anyone who has a family history of alcoholism or binge drinking should check with their physician before using alcohol. Alcohol is not recommended for pregnant women.

Please note that I recommend that magnesium and carnitine be taken twice a day, the other ingredients of the Elixir only once a day. They also can be taken twice a day, however, to make it easier for you to remember—more specifically, you may take 200 international units of vitamin E, 200 micrograms of folic acid, 200 to 250 milligrams of vitamin B_6, and 250 to 500 micrograms of vitamin B_{12} twice a day.

No exact formula for the Cardiac Elixir presently exists for you to purchase. You must, therefore, make a special effort on your own to find the proper formulations that contain the recommended doses.

CHAPTER SEVEN

Carnitine: The Centerpiece of the Elixir

Carnitine is the world's best-kept nutraceutical secret. There are numerous well-conducted clinical studies that clearly demonstrate its beneficial effects both in treating patients with heart disease and in preventing heart disease. Carnitine can protect the heart muscle against ischemia, or reduced bloodflow, and cellular damage caused by lack of oxygen. But despite the strong evidence from clinical studies, carnitine has not received the media attention of other nutraceuticals for which the clinical experimental evidence is far less powerful.

But carnitine's day is coming.

It's inevitable, because clinical data—studies actually done in real live human beings—are the driving force of the nutraceutical revolution, and the carnitine results are just too positive to be overlooked much longer.

I'll never forget Anna, a young Florida woman with an undiagnosed heart ailment who clung to life on a respirator. The standard medical treatment hadn't helped her. But she responded dramatically to carnitine.

I also have vivid memories of a newborn at Bethesda Naval Hospital in Maryland who couldn't move his arms or legs, couldn't even suckle, until he was given carnitine; and of 9-year old Marina, who was awaiting death from a congenital heart disease that had already claimed the lives of her three siblings, before carnitine therapy saved her life.

It's important to understand that these seeming miraculous effects involved people who had serious heart problems due to a rare type of profound carnitine deficiency. It's most common among infants and children whose bodies have failed to develop the ability to synthesize adequate amounts of carnitine. However, the carnitine deficiency that we'll be talking about isn't a systemwide deficiency, but a deficiency in the heart—either a part or most of the organ. The heart requires higher levels of carnitine than most of the tissues of the body.

I don't want to create the impression that carnitine is a miracle fix for a person with atherosclerosis or coronary heart disease. This is not the case. Proper use of carnitine as part of the Cardiac Elixir, however, adds to your chances of achieving optimal cardiac health. The best medical evidence strongly suggests that supplementation with carnitine can keep your heart pumping strongly, help fight the onset of heart disease, and, perhaps most important, protect you in the event you do have a heart attack.

The plain fact is that even people who do everything right—who eat properly, exercise, relax, and use supplements wisely—are stricken with heart attacks. Carnitine is a heart attack insurance policy. There is compelling evidence that high levels of carnitine in your system can minimize damage to the heart muscle that takes place during a heart attack. Carnitine supplements offer an effective one-two punch. They can help keep your heart healthy and protect it during a cardiac crisis.

The Energy-Making Molecule

Carnitine is not an amino acid as often advertised. It is instead manufactured by our liver and kidneys out of two amino acids, lysine and methionine, into what is called a quaternary amine. It's found in some foods, including meats, fish, and dairy products. Carnitine's most important role in our bodies is to get fuel into our cells, specifically, the part of the cell called the mitochondria. The mitochondria can be thought of as the cellular furnace. They turn the fuel in food into energy or ATP (adenosine triphosphate), the energy molecule.

Our bodies have two primary sources of fuel: sugar and fatty acids. The metabolism of fat produces roughly twice as much en-

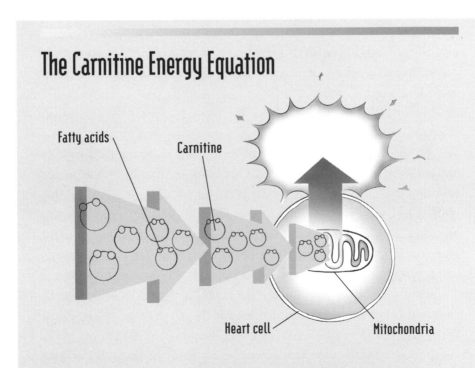

The Carnitine Energy Equation

Fatty acids

Carnitine

Heart cell

Mitochondria

Carnitine molecules escort fatty acids through the outer mitochondrial membranes found in heart cells so that fatty acids can be converted to energy.

ergy as sugar. Since the heart is constantly at work, even when we're resting, it requires an enormous amount of energy to sustain itself. Fatty acids are the cardiac fuel of choice.

Carnitine is so important for cardiac health because without it, fatty acids can't cross into the mitochondrial furnace. The carnitine molecule escorts the fatty acids through the outer mitochondrial membrane so that they can be turned into energy.

In the absence of carnitine, fatty acids can't get in. If our hearts can't get fatty acids, they turn, in an emergency, to sugar as a backup fuel.

But sugar often does not provide enough energy for the heart to keep beating regularly. In many cases, severe arrhythmias can lead to cardiac arrest and death.

Carnitine is the stoker, the molecule that shovels fuel into the engine. It makes cardiac energy possible. In a way, the onset of heart disease is a process of energy starvation. If your heart doesn't get enough high-quality fuel, it can't produce enough energy to pump blood to the rest of your body tissues as well as to sustain itself.

Here's what happens when your heart doesn't get enough oxygen.

When the amount of oxygen—remember, the blood carries oxygen—available to your heart cells is diminished, the outer membrane of the myocardial cells become more porous. When this happens, carnitine leaks out of the heart cells and back into the bloodstream. When the carnitine leaks out, the fatty acids can't cross the mitochondrial membrane to be metabolized. This results in an energy crisis. The heart's pumping ability is diminished.

Also, on top of the energy shortage, a shortage of carnitine causes another problem. Since there's little or no carnitine to carry them into the mitochondria, fatty acids build up in the cardiac cells. Unused fatty acids can themselves be toxic to heart cells and can contribute to arrhythmias and even cell death.

Supplemental carnitine can prevent this downward spiral by keeping carnitine levels up in spite of the leakage caused by oxygen deprivation.

The Early Studies: How Carnitine Helps the Ischemic Struggling Heart

The first steps on the path to the Carnitine Defense were studies that explored how carnitine could help the heart that was already compromised. Way back in 1966, after an early, small clinical study, an unexpected finding led me to believe that carnitine may be able to protect the heart against myocardial ischemia, reduced bloodflow to the heart. I turned excitedly to the medical literature to see what I could find about carnitine and the heart.

The physiological role of carnitine had been studied in the 1930s and 1940s. That early study, conducted with rats, showed the important role that carnitine played in the transport of fatty acids. At that time, there had been no studies in people to support the idea of carnitine's cardiac benefit. But I postulated that carnitine could help people with myocardial ischemia, whether or not they had had a heart attack. The reasoning was simple and straightforward. Remember the patient in my hyperthyroid study that I described in chapter 1? He had told me that carnitine gave him relief from angina pain that he had endured for 20 years. Interestingly enough, if it weren't for that one man, scientific and medical research on the cardiac benefits of carnitine could have been delayed for a very long time.

The medical experts I consulted were skeptical. They logically argued that if the heart cells were already damaged by lack of oxygen, giving them more energy through carnitine supplementation would only make them work harder and create more cell damage. But it seemed to me that the consistent positive findings of the early animal studies overrode the theoretical concerns of the experts. My readings in the literature, combined with some encouragement from a few cardiologist colleagues, further convinced me that carnitine could indeed help patients with ischemia. I was eager to move forward with clinical trials giving carnitine to patients with cardiovascular disease.

The effort was interrupted by a call from Uncle Sam. I was

A Superb Safety Record

Carnitine is both safe and effective. Because it is available in prescription form, and doctors have to report any negative side effects, the data on carnitine's safety are far more compelling than most other natural substances. Prescription carnitine has been given to nearly one million people worldwide, and there has been no evidence of significant side effects. One reason why carnitine supplementation is safe is that carnitine is a water-soluble molecule, which means that the body doesn't store it up. If you have more than you can use, it simply gets excreted through urination.

By way of absolutely full disclosure, I should say that occasionally, a very small percentage of people report mild nausea or diarrhea when they begin carnitine supplementation. Most often, these unusual side effects disappear as your body gets used to the carnitine. However, if these side effects persist or worsen, talk to your doctor.

Before you start taking carnitine or any supplement, talk to your doctor about it. It's important to review the other medications or supplements that you may be taking. Tell your doctor and pharmacist about all other prescription drugs, over-the-counter products, and dietary supplements that you're taking. The more knowledge of your habits your doctor has, the better care he or she can provide.

drafted to serve in the Vietnam War. Fortunately, I was spared combat when a computer, searching for a drug expert, came upon my training in clinical pharmacology. Clinical pharmacology is the medical speciality that deals with testing substances in people to determine whether they have a medical benefit. I was assigned to the Walter Reed Army Institute of Research in Washington, D.C., to head up a unit doing clinical research into drugs that had shown promise in animal studies. The government was specifically looking for anti-malarial and anti-radiation compounds.

At the time, I was disappointed that I couldn't pursue my carnitine research. But my stint at Walter Reed turned out to be one of life's serendipitous blessings. It was and remains a first-class medical institution, and I was lucky enough to convince Major James Vick, Ph.D., an influential and energetic cardiac pharmacologist, that carnitine was worth exploring.

We undertook a long series of animal studies spearheaded by Major Vick. Since our research had little direct military application, we did most of our experiments after hours. The results were eye-opening.

We found that carnitine gave dramatic protection to animal hearts. And we found this protective effect under many different stressed conditions. Carnitine helped animal hearts deal with toxins, bacteria, even snake venom in test after test. Whether in isolated heart models or in living animals, we observed that carnitine could minimize the negative effects of decreased oxygen availability to the heart.

Some Setbacks—And Then a Breakthrough

The exciting test results we got in our animal studies only made me more determined to move forward to trials on people. But I had virtually no financial support. Drug companies were just not interested in funding studies with weakly patented natural substances such as carnitine. (As we saw in chapter 3, drug companies seek strong patents on artificial molecules so they can totally own and market them without any threat of competition. Carnitine and other natural substances can only be protected through limited patent protection, such as for a unique dosage formulation.)

Because it was very expensive to conduct these trials in the United States, I decided to do them overseas. My hope was that if I got some promising results in foreign countries, I would be able to get U.S. funding. In the meantime, I borrowed money from the bank in order to keep the carnitine project going.

At the suggestion of my friend, James Rand, an independent creative medical entrepreneur, I went to Germany and met with

Secrets of the Mitochondria— and Other Uses of Carnitine

There has been an explosive growth in the study of mitochondria. This area of research promises to improve our understanding and treatment of disease tremendously. While the jury is not yet in, I think it's safe to say that the mitochondria will be found to play a crucial role in a great number of chronic diseases, such as Alzheimer's, Parkinson's, cancer, diabetes, and heart disease. And carnitine is inextricably bound up in optimal mitochondrial functioning.

I think it's likely that this exciting research into the mitochondria will bring carnitine to the fore in connection with many diseases. Already, there are several other medical conditions in which carnitine plays a valuable role.

Renal dialysis. Studies of more than 1,000 patients show that carnitine dramatically helps patients on kidney (or renal) dialysis who are weak, have muscle cramps, and whose quality of life is poor.

Male infertility. Infertility is often associated with a condition called male sperm hypomotility. The sperm tail doesn't have enough energy to wiggle with enough vigor to get to the waiting egg. Researchers have discovered that, generally, these sperm are carnitine-deficient. In Europe, clinical studies have shown that the administration of carnitine significantly increases both the motility of sperm and the sperm count.

AIDS. People with AIDS have a marked decrease in carnitine levels. In addition, AIDS patients experience dramatic increases in the death of virus-fighting white blood cells. Studies have shown that carnitine inhibits this process.

Hyperthyroidism. People with hyperthyroidism have an overactive thy-

the owner of a large pharmaceutical firm, Dr. Rolf Madaus, and made my case. He graciously gave me enough money to continue my preclinical studies and begin a clinical trial in Yugoslavia.

It was not my finest hour. In Phase I, we set out to determine if our dosage formulation was safe. But from the beginning, we ran roid, which produces too much thyroid hormone. I did a clinical study way back in 1965 showing that carnitine is effective in managing this condition. How can carnitine do this when we know that it did not—and does not—block thyroid hormone production? My theory was that the thyroid hormone might well accentuate the activity of another hormone, adrenalin, which is a stimulant and increases the body's metabolism. Carnitine might be able to block adrenalin's effect and thereby improve the patient's hyperthyroid signs and symptoms. But truthfully, we simply don't know.

Rare metabolic disorders. There is a lot of evidence that carnitine deficiency causes a number of rare disorders, such as cardiomyopathy in children, that can be successfully managed with carnitine.

Toxicity. In many animal studies, carnitine has prevented deaths and reversed the damage from toxicity caused by a wide range of substances, such as antidepressants, beta blockers, *E. coli*, and snake venom. Carnitine helped preserve a functioning cardiovascular system, reverse toxicity, and prevent death.

Adriamycin cardiac toxicity. Adriamycin is an effective anti-cancer drug, but its dose often has to be limited because it can cause heart failure. On top of this, the early phases of adriamycin administration frequently cause acute effects, such as abnormal changes in peoples' electrocardiograms as well as increases in their blood cardiac enzymes, which reflect heart cell damage. We know that carnitine decreases both these acute effects in humans. We also know that carnitine blocks the chronic heart toxicity problem in animals. Studies on the effect of carnitine on the long–term or chronic toxicity in humans, which is admittedly more important, have not yet been done. Carnitine blocks this chronic toxicity in animal studies as well as in the early phases of toxicity in humans.

into problems, starting with the difficulty of producing the intravenous form of carnitine. One of the researchers temporarily lost his sight while sterilizing the carnitine with ultraviolet light in the laboratory. Other physician-researchers, using highly concentrated intravenous carnitine, came down with serious phlebitis after using themselves as human experimental subjects. Eventually, an associate and I injected ourselves with a diluted version of carnitine, and when no phlebitis occurred, we proceeded with this dosage formulation.

These early clinical trials did little to advance the cause of carnitine as a medicine. We tested carnitine as a therapy for a few selected diseases, but the initial trial showed no clear-cut activity. Even in patients with ischemia and congestive heart failure, carnitine appeared to have no dramatic therapeutic effect.

Given what has been discovered since those early trials about carnitine's benefits to people with heart disease, I can only assume that the early studies were either badly designed or poorly executed. This is not a criticism of the physicians who did the trials. They were all competent and sincere. Indeed, I approved the clinical protocols. But in those early days of carnitine research, we were all groping a bit, trying to find our way. The discouraging results were probably the result of using a faulty formulation of intravenous carnitine, the wrong dose, or of timing the duration of its administration incorrectly.

After this setback, I wanted to develop an oral dose of carnitine. But once again, funding was a problem. The cost of developing carnitine that could be taken by mouth, and meet U.S. government guidelines, was staggering. I found an American pharmaceutical company that paid for some preliminary clinical trials in the United States, but once again, the results were not dramatic, and the company canceled its support of the clinical trials.

Even I was beginning to doubt carnitine. Throughout those difficult days, I was sustained by those early animal studies and the enthusiasm of Major Vick at Walter Reed. Every time I began to lose faith in carnitine's potential, I thought of those dramatic animal experiment results. Surely, I thought, if carnitine could have such a clear-cut effect on compromised animal hearts, it must be able to protect human hearts as well.

But my optimism and even my reasoning could have been faulty. Many effects in animals are not translatable into humans. I decided to keep going forward, but by the mid 1970s, I was in carnitine limbo, uncertain about what to do next. Then another lucky break came my way.

I met Austin Shug, Ph.D., a scientist at the University of Wisconsin. Dr. Shug was a respected scientist who, unbeknownst to me, had already conducted a number of studies of carnitine in animal models. His work went a step beyond those studies that we had done at Walter Reed. In one, he subjected animal hearts to the same ischemic damage that occurs during a heart attack. Dr. Shug discovered a markedly lower concentration of carnitine only in the ischemic area of the heart. He also found, over time, a correlation between the loss of carnitine in this area of the heart and cardiac damage. Most important, he found that by administering carnitine before or during the time when the animal hearts were deprived of oxygen, he could prevent or reverse damaging ischemic changes. Carnitine enabled the animal heart in crisis to use its fatty acids more efficiently and function more normally.

Dr. Shug introduced me to his medical colleague, James Thomsen, M.D., a cardiologist, to discuss initiating trials in people in the United States. Dr. Thomsen suggested that we parallel Dr. Shug's animal studies as closely as possible in humans. We initiated a clinical trial of carnitine on people with myocardial ischemia. Generally speaking, these patients often suffer from plaques in their coronary arteries. When these plaques keep blood from flowing freely to the heart, the result is frequently chest pain. Their electrocardiograms, or EKGs, and blood tests usually show changes in the heart's electrical conduction and in enzyme levels that are typical of a stressed heart.

In his clinical study, Dr. Thomsen used a technique called atrial pacing. This is a medical diagnostic procedure that helps doctors evaluate the seriousness of ischemic heart disease. A catheter is inserted into a vein and then guided carefully to the heart. At this point, the heart is electrically stimulated to make it beat faster, thereby increasing its need for energy. Because the heart is working harder, the patient will eventually experience chest pain or display other cardiac changes, such as EKG changes that indicate insufficient bloodflow and oxygen supply to the heart. Doctors can tell the extent of the ischemic heart disease by observing when the chest pain begins and when the abnormal changes in the EKG appear.

Dr. Thomsen gave half of the patients carnitine and the others a placebo. His findings were positive. The hearts of the patients who had been given carnitine worked longer before they had chest pain or other signs of diminished bloodflow to the heart. This study was a landmark in carnitine research. It was the very first clinical trial to show that carnitine could minimize the damaging effects of myocardial ischemia.

Elated by the findings of Dr. Shug and Dr. Thomsen, I then assembled a group of the world's top medical experts to review the data. I wanted to be sure that my own eagerness to believe in carnitine wasn't clouding my judgment concerning the results of the studies. The physician-experts concluded that Dr. Thomsen's study indeed supported the effectiveness of carnitine in the prevention of myocardial ischemia. When the paper about Dr. Thomsen's study was published in the prestigious *American Journal of Cardiology*, it was a milestone in the investigation of the medical promise of carnitine for ischemic heart disease.

The Carnitine Evidence Builds

Since this first important study, the clinical evidence on behalf of carnitine has continued to grow. Dr. Thomsen did another clinical study using the treadmill instead of atrial pacing. It, too, showed that carnitine improved the myocardial metabolism of patients with ischemic heart disease and helped them perform more efficiently. In the years since, many other studies—including very convincing clinical pharmacologic studies—have supported and expanded Dr. Thomsen's early conclusions.

A clinical pharmacologic study is one in which the patient is studied and closely monitored in the hospital itself. Unlike epidemiological studies—which are based on statistical analysis of large

groups and the results of which can be equivocal or not definitive—well-conducted clinical pharmacologic studies are rarely
questioned by physicians.

All in all, there have been eight clinical pharmacologic studies
that demonstrated carnitine's beneficial effect in patients with coronary artery disease and myocardial ischemia. The ischemic hearts
were stressed by either atrial pacing or exercise. The studies demonstrated that carnitine enhanced the metabolism of heart cells and
helped hearts perform more efficiently.

In 1991, Carl Pepine, M.D., professor of medicine and co-
director of the division of cardiology at the University of Florida
in Gainesville, published a review of the clinical research on carnitine in *Clinical Therapeutics*. He found that these studies reported
that carnitine improved the exercise capacity of heart patients as
well as their EKG results and their heart function.

I know of no other cardiac nutraceutical that has been put to
this extensive clinical testing in patients with myocardial ischemia.

Help for the Heart Attack Victim

Following up on the clinical pharmacologic studies that
demonstrated carnitine's anti-ischemic activity, a small pilot study
was conducted on patients who had heart attacks and were hos-
pitalized within 8 hours of the onset of chest pain. For the first
5 days, carnitine was administered along with standard drugs that
physicians use to minimize cardiac damage and increase the
chances of survival. A biomarker, or substance that is present in
the blood to measure damage or dead myocardial cells called
MB-CPK, was measured both in the patients who received carnitine and those that did not. Generally, the biomarker indicating
cell damage was significantly lower in the group that received
carnitine.

Another study was conducted in patients with coronary artery
disease who underwent bypass surgery. Twenty patients were given
carnitine before and during surgery. A control group of 20 patients

Sigma Tau: A Pillar of Support for Carnitine

Fortune smiled on me and patients everywhere when, in 1978, I met Claudio Cavazza, Ph.D., the owner and president of Sigma Tau, a pharmaceutical company based in Pomezia, Italy, and a strong advocate of carnitine research.

When I met Dr. Cavazza, I had already been to 33 other companies in my search for a firm willing to license carnitine and encountered strong resistance. Dr. Cavazza responded with immediate and vigorous support. He is one of the few leaders in the pharmaceutical and other health industries that I have met who truly understands medicine and science. Because of this understanding, he has devoted his energies to developing carnitine as a pharmaceutical drug. By sponsoring many clinical studies in the United States and throughout the world, he continues to demonstrate carnitine's clinical benefits in many diseases. Thanks to his efforts, he has encouraged his company, Sigma Tau, to manufacture and sell carnitine either by itself or through licensing agreements with other companies all over the world, including in the United States.

did not receive carnitine. The results showed that the ATP or energy storage concentrations in the heart muscle of the carnitine group was significantly higher. Also, the lactate concentrations were much lower in this group. Lactate is a waste product that builds up if fatty acids are not burning efficiently. It is an indicator of lack of oxygen. So a low level of lactate indicates more healthy myocardial metabolism.

In an extensive multicenter, double-blind study conducted in Italy and the Netherlands, researchers gave carnitine intravenously to half of the people who were admitted to the hospital within a short time after the beginning of a heart attack. The carnitine group continued to receive carnitine in pill form for a year after the heart attack. The other half of the patients in the study received a placebo.

The researchers evaluated the patients by looking at the left ventricular wall of their hearts. A healthy left ventricle is essential to maintain the pumping efficiency of the heart. If a heart attack destroys enough of the muscle in this area, the heart becomes incapable of pumping normally. The results of the study, published in 1995 in the *Journal of the American College of Clinical Cardiology*, showed that more ventricular heart muscle survived in the patients who were given carnitine. The interpretation of this finding meant that the heart could pump more efficiently because carnitine decreased cell death that occurred due to a lack of oxygen.

A similar double-blind clinical trial, conducted by R. B. Singh, affiliated with the Heart Research Laboratory and Centre of Nutrition Research at the Medical Hospital and Research Centre in Moradabad, India, and his colleagues and published in the *Postgraduate Medical Journal*, supported the results of the European study. Each patient, all of whom were admitted to the hospital after the onset of a heart attack, was given either carnitine or a placebo for 28 days starting right after their heart attacks. The clinical researchers concluded that patients on carnitine had a significantly smaller area of heart tissue damaged by the attack. They also had lower blood levels of disease-associated lipids as well as fewer arrhythmias. The placebo group had twice as many deaths and second heart attacks as the carnitine group.

Another study, involving patients who had a second heart attack, used a different technique for measuring the protective effect of carnitine. With his colleagues, K. G. C. Jacoba, affiliated with the Philippine Heart Center in Quezon Citya, Philippines, used a sophisticated imaging camera to take pictures of the heart muscles of the patients every 2 weeks, both before and after exercise on a treadmill. The patients all took either carnitine or a placebo for 8 weeks starting a month after their heart attacks. The physician-researchers reported that the images showed that those who took carnitine had more heart muscle left and less dead tissue than the placebo-treated patients. This is an especially promising study in that it showed that carnitine can work on the damaged, compromised cells that don't die during a heart attack even when carnitine is administered a month afterward, and it can help bring them back to normal. Carnitine also may help prevent the death of damaged heart cells that are compromised, struggling to survive, and would eventually die in the absence of high levels of carnitine.

Are You on the Path to Ischemia?

All this talk of studies on patients with myocardial ischemia and patients who have had heart attacks may leave you thinking, "What about me?" After all, you don't have ischemia, and your heart is in good shape, right?

Maybe.

I don't mean to be an alarmist, but a case can be made that, from our youth, we're all on the path to heart disease. You know the old bromide that middle age just sort of sneaks up on you. One minute, you're 22, and before you know it, you're 45. There's no clearly definable moment at which you become middle-aged; it's an eventuality that happens a day at a time. Many medical diseases, including heart disease, involve the same the same kind of incremental process.

A thought-provoking study on autopsied solders killed in the Korean War reported that many of those men—in their twenties or even their teens—had the beginnings of atherosclerosis. Deposits had built up inside their blood vessels. Another study, done by Jack P. Strong, M.D., chairman of pathology at the Louisiana State University Medical Center in New Orleans and reported in the *Journal of the American Medical Association* in 1999, revealed that the process of arterial plaque buildup can materialize as early as age 15.

When the bloodflow to our hearts is greatly compromised, we usually have signs and symptoms, most often the chest pain known as angina pectoris. Once we have the pain of angina, we know that heart cells are being damaged by a lack of oxygen.

What medical science doesn't know is how much cellular damage occurs before these signs and symptoms appear. In other words, how small a reduction in bloodflow can undermine the condition of a particular individual's heart cells?

The onset of most ischemic heart disease is gradual, involving the microscopic narrowing of coronary arteries. But there can sometimes be as much as a 40 percent or more blockage in bloodflow before there are cardiac symptoms. And, most important concerning carnitine supplementation, there is evidence to suggest that long before symptoms appear, heart cells die.

Many people who have significant ischemia don't get nature's warning signal, anginal chest pain. They have what's known as silent ischemia. Though exactly how many people have the sneaky version of ischemia is hard to determine, it's not unreasonable to assume that they number in the many millions. Beyond that, even if in strict medical terms you can't be classified as having ischemia, a large majority of people have a gradual narrowing of the arteries as they age.

A Carnitine Profile

What it is:
A natural proteinlike substance found in some foods and manufactured in our liver and kidneys from two amino acids

What it does:
Transports fatty acids, a source of fuel for the body, into heart cells

Mechanism of protection:
Your heart cells turn fatty acids into the energy they need to say alive and keep beating

Where you can buy it:
Pharmacies, health food stores, and some supermarkets; in capsule, tablet, and liquid form; also available by prescription

What to look for on the label:
L-carnitine

Who it's for:
Adults over age 35, especially those in certain high-risk categories

How much to take:
1,500 to 3,000 milligrams daily, divided into two doses, 8 to 12 hours apart.

Here's why I think carnitine supplements are an important part of optimal heart health.

There is overwhelming evidence that carnitine can help the compromised heart. And since in many people, it's nearly impossible to know whether or not our hearts are compromised, it makes good medical sense to take carnitine. It can help prevent or minimize cardiac cell damage that might result from even the earliest stages of coronary artery blockage. Carnitine supplementation is an effective, natural way of protecting your heart. Especially when taken along with the other supplements in the Cardiac Elixir, carnitine reduces the risk of cardiac crisis.

Who Should Take Carnitine?

Should everybody take carnitine supplements?

Most physicians, including me, tend to resist sweeping statements. There are so many variables in everybody's medical history that it's often unwise to make generalizations. But that said, I'm tempted to get somewhat dogmatic about carnitine. Based on animal and clinical studies, the medical evidence is extremely strong. I believe that most people over age 35 should take carnitine supplements. It can help prevent or reduce the cellular damage associated with ischemia. Further, since we're all at some risk of heart attack, it makes sense to keep our carnitine levels high.

During a heart attack, your body needs more carnitine than ever to enter back into heart cells and combat the life-threatening crisis. The normal blood levels of carnitine are just not high enough. Carnitine supplementation can actually normalize the functioning of cardiac cells when the blood supply to the heart is inadequate. The plain fact is that coronary artery disease can develop without symptoms. For many, sudden death may be the first and last warning sign.

Based on the clinical evidence, here are some specific recommendations for people who can benefit from carnitine supplementation. As you'll see, these groups, taken together, include a great many of us. Plenty of perfectly healthy people should make carnitine part of their daily routines, including:

- *People who have a family history of heart disease*
- *People who are overweight*
- *People with high blood pressure*
- *People with high cholesterol*
- *People with diabetes*

In addition, people who have heart disease, particularly those with myocardial ischemia, can benefit from boosting their carnitine levels in several ways.

People who have had heart attacks should take supplements of carnitine. There is overwhelming evidence that carnitine can protect heart cells that lack oxygen. The data also demonstrate that carnitine supplementation can limit subsequent cellular damage that may lead to a second heart attack.

People over age 40 who exercise may benefit from taking carnitine before exercise. It may help protect your heart from any damaging ischemia related to strenuous exertion.

People who have cardiomyopathy due to myocardial ischemia may need carnitine. In general, cardiomyopathy is the name for a weakened heart muscle that causes reduced heart contractions and decreased blood circulation to the lungs and the rest of the body. Cardiomyopathy patients usually feel fatigued and often have chest pain. Many experience abnormal heart rhythms such as atrial fibrillation, which are rapid, irregular contractions of the upper chambers of the heart. The reduction in the heart's pumping capacity for patients with cardiomyopathy can be so significant that it leads to congestive heart failure, which causes breathing difficulty and swelling in the hands and legs. For many such people, the heart continues to deteriorate, and a heart transplant is the only option.

What causes cardiomyopathy? Many such patients have what is

known as idiopathic cardiomyopathy, which means that the cause is unknown. Theoretically, carnitine should benefit these people, but the clinical studies needed to adequately test this possibility have not yet been done.

On the other hand, a significant number of patients have cardiomyopathy due to myocardial ischemia, which results in heart attacks that destroy large amounts of heart muscle. This is known as ischemic cardiomyopathy. In these cases, clinical studies indicate that carnitine can play a significant role in preventing the progress of this condition.

An estimated four million people in the United States have either idiopathic or ischemic cardiomyopathy.

How You Should Use Carnitine

Carnitine is the keystone of the Cardiac Elixir. It is essential that you use a carnitine product that is safe and effective and that provides you with the maximum protection that carnitine can offer your heart. The information below will help you do just that.

Though carnitine is a simple molecule, it's a hard molecule to work with. So for packaging purposes, it has to be combined with another molecule, usually a salt. There are basically four chemical formulations of carnitine. One is an FDA-approved pharmaceutical product available only by prescription. Three dietary supplement formulations are freely available for purchase in drugstores and health food stores: L-carnitine hydrochloride, L-carnitine tartrate, and L-carnitine fumarate. These formulations are available in tablet, capsule, or liquid. Though all three dietary forms will give you heart protection, the best bet is carnitine fumurate. Here's why.

Carnitine fumurate enters the body more easily than the other formulations. Fumaric acid, or fumarate, is a naturally occurring substance in the body that enters the energy cycle within the mitochondria and has the potential to help provide your body with

The Quality of Supplements

Given the explosion in the world of supplements, it's not always easy to be sure that you're getting high-quality products. Some companies put out supplements of inferior quality.

You should always check with your doctor before taking carnitine, but don't overlook your pharmacist as a good source of information about the reliability of the company making the carnitine supplement—or any supplement, for that matter. Pharmacists are important and knowledgeable allies for consumers, and they're trained to educate people about over-the-counter products. Keep in mind, however, that because of the newness of the Nutraceutical Revolution, pharmacists are like most of us—only beginning to learn about dietary supplements.

more energy. Fumarate also functions as an antioxidant and free radical scavenger.

Many studies have shown that fumarate itself helps protect heart muscle cells damaged by ischemia. In animal studies, researchers found that the addition of carnitine fumarate to the standard blood solution was much better than the standard solution alone in bringing about the improved functional recovery of the heart. In an animal study involving isolated rat hearts that were deprived of oxygen, researchers discovered that fumarate improved the functioning of the left ventricle of the heart.

Researchers at Georgetown University Medical Center in Washington, D.C., conducted an experiment to determine whether carnitine fumarate salt is superior to carnitine alone in protecting the ischemic heart. They found that carnitine fumarate was superior to carnitine alone in preserving high–ATP energy levels and in decreasing levels of lactate production (a standard sign of ischemia) by the heart. The researchers concluded that there was a clearly demonstrated synergistic effect of carnitine and fumarate that was even more effective than carnitine alone in protecting against myocardial ischemia.

In conclusion, scientific studies consistently report that both carnitine and fumarate individually protect against myocardial ischemia. Working together, they appear to have a benefit greater than either one alone. It seems logical, therefore, that the combination of carnitine and fumarate would offer significant advantages over other carnitine salts, all of which lack fumarate's beneficial effects.

It has been difficult for consumers to tell which kind of carnitine they were getting because manufacturers were not required to specify the formulation on the label. But law now mandates that all products manufactured after March 1999 indicate on the label which kind of carnitine is being used. So if the product that you're considering doesn't say what kind of carnitine is being used, don't buy it. Look for the words "L-carnitine fumarate" on the label.

How Much Carnitine Should You Take?

Though the body makes its own carnitine, it doesn't make enough to give you optimal heart protection. Nor can you get enough from your diet. Carnitine is available in meat, chicken, fish, and dairy products, but only in small amounts. Further, your body can only absorb about 25 percent of the carnitine that it gets through your diet. I cannot stress this enough: No matter what you eat and how much carnitine your body is able to make, you need to take carnitine supplements to protect your heart, especially under high-stress conditions.

Clinical studies suggest that you should take 1,500 to 3,000 milligrams of carnitine a day. I prefer the higher dose, but it is rather expensive.

Considered in purely biological terms, the liquid form may be best. It enters the bloodstream more quickly, and more may be absorbed by the body. But liquid carnitine has a downside. It tends to taste bitter. Try it to see how you respond to it. Most people prefer using the capsules or tablets.

In addition to tablets, capsules, and liquid, carnitine may soon be available in the form of a powder that dissolves when you place it in a liquid. Generally speaking, putting carnitine into liquid formulation increases the possibility of better absorption by the body.

To make sure that you don't forget your carnitine, take it with meals or just after meals. Try to take your dose of carnitine at regular times each day, with at least 8 to 12 hours between doses. Carnitine achieves its best effects when a constant amount is maintained in the blood.

If you miss a dose, it isn't necessary to double up your dosage. Simply skip the missed dosage and continue on with your regular schedule of carnitine supplementation.

CHAPTER EIGHT

Vitamin E and Healthy Arteries

Like much of what we know about natural substances, the medical story of vitamin E began with research on laboratory rats. Back in 1922, researchers at the University of California were trying to isolate a substance in wheat germ that appeared to help the rodents reproduce. They eventually came upon a gold-colored chemical that they named factor X.

Two years later, researchers at the University of Arkansas rechristened factor X "vitamin E." And later still, tipping their hats toward vitamin E's fertility function, scientists began referring to it as tocopherol, from the Greek words *tokos* meaning "offspring" and *pherein* meaning "to bear." For a while, we didn't learn much more about this yellowish fatty chemical.

But then, in the 1940s, two Canadian physicians, brothers named Evan and Wilfrid Shute, put forth the theory that vitamin E could help fight heart disease.

They didn't get far with this idea. Their ideas were controversial and met resistance from doctors and other researchers. But for-

110

tunately, the Shute brothers kept plugging away. They noticed a drastic rise in the number of heart failure cases, which they believed coincided with a decision by the food-processing industry to eliminate wheat germ—high in vitamin E—from white flour during the milling process. When the Shutes had no luck getting their findings published in a medical journal, they just started their own, *The Summary*.

Since those early controversial days, vitamin E has become one of the most widely researched nutrients. There is some evidence that it may be useful in helping treat or prevent a wide variety of diseases.

But the evidence on behalf of vitamin E as a cardiovascular nutraceutical is already compelling. The research results in favor of vitamin E have been developing for years.

In the early 1980s, early studies—like most preliminary medical research done on laboratory animals—showed that both rodents and piglets whose diets were deficient in vitamin E were prone to atherosclerosis. When the animals were given extra vitamin E, the amount of arterial plaque decreased. Indeed, a well-designed study by a team from the University of Pittsburgh published in *Nature* in 1998 found that mice given vitamin E for 16 weeks had 40 percent less plaque in their arteries than mice who had not been given vitamin E.

Before exploring the research in humans, which further supports the importance of vitamin E supplements, let's take a look at the mechanism of nutraceutical protection, how experts believe vitamin E protects us.

How Vitamin E Defuses Plaque Time Bombs

Vitamin E's greatest benefit is that it can help neutralize the most dangerous form of cholesterol—low-density lipoproteins (LDLs)—before and even after they can start plaque formation in your arteries.

Your blood carries the fats needed by every cell of your body

Vitamin E's Versatility: Other Nutraceutical Possibilities

Because damage caused by free radicals contributes to many disease conditions, and vitamin E is such a powerful antioxidant, lots of health claims are made for supplements of vitamin E. In my opinion, many of them are premature or even misleading. But there's no question in my mind that vitamin E is a versatile nutraceutical and will be proven to help prevent or manage many other health problems.

Though the research is at an early stage, here are a few of the conditions for which vitamin E may indeed be helpful.

Diabetes. Vitamin E may be especially useful to people with diabetes because their arteries tend to develop plaque more than in people who don't have diabetes. And it's entirely possible that people with diabetes experience the bad effects of free radicals more than others. Vitamin E also may reduce the resistance to insulin to which people with diabetes are prone. In addition, vitamin E seems to improve the ability to tolerate glucose for people with diabetes.

Age-related impaired immunity. Researchers at Tufts University in Medford, Massachusetts, Harvard University, and Boston University supple-

in the form of lipoproteins—large fat particles encased in proteins that make the fats soluble in your blood. High-density lipoproteins, or HDLs, carry the so-called "good" cholesterol from your arteries to special HDL receptors in your liver, which facilitate cholesterol breakdown and secretion, or else they store it safely for later use. Your low-density lipoproteins, on the other hand, carry the "bad" cholesterol to your arteries. These are the big threat to your cardiovascular health. They can turn into plaque.

The process by which LDL turns into plaque is complex. It starts when electrons get knocked off oxygen molecules in your blood, creating molecules called free radicals. These free radicals are mented the diets of 88 people older than age 65 with vitamin E. They found that a daily dose of 200 international units (IU) improved immunity by 65 percent, judging from the skin sensitivity that indicates immune response. They also found that the vitamin E produced a sixfold increase in antibodies against the one infectious disease that they tested for: hepatitis B. Other studies on immunity have found that older folks who took supplements had 30 percent fewer bouts with colds, flu, and pneumonia. Whether vitamin E boosts younger immune systems is yet to be studied.

Alzheimer's disease. Researchers now think that vitamin E's antioxidant effect seems to slow down the signs and symptoms of Alzheimer's disease. A clinical trial, including more than 300 people across the United States and published in the *New England Journal of Medicine* in 1998, found that 2,000 IU of vitamin E daily had a significant effect on the lives of people with Alzheimer's. They were able to take care of themselves longer and were able to delay their entry into nursing homes. Though memory didn't improve, the evidence of a benefit was strong enough to compel the American Psychiatric Association to include a recommendation for vitamin E supplements in its latest guidelines. This is a very high dose of vitamin E and should only be taken under the close supervision of a physician.

as unstable as hormonal teenagers. They roam your bloodstream in search of the electron that they're missing. That's where the LDLs come in. The pillaging free radicals glom onto them in search of the electron that they lack. The resultant LDL-oxygen union is a formula for artery trouble.

LDLs in combination with oxygen are especially atherogenic. That's a fancy term that means they start the process of plaque formation. Once your LDLs get oxidized, they become a multifaceted threat to your heart health. Here's the series of bad-news cardiovascular events that take place once LDL and oxygen get paired.

1. The "marriage" attracts the attention of your white blood cells, which normally circulate freely throughout your blood to fight off bacteria and viruses. Some of these white blood cells become transformed into macrophages, which are white blood cells responsible for engulfing and ingesting bacteria and other microscopic invaders. These macrophages react to the merged LDL-oxygen molecule as an invader. They begin building up and sticking to the cells lining your artery walls.

How Plaque Forms in an Artery

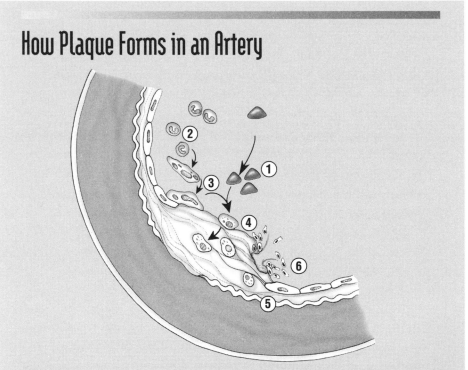

As LDL-oxygen molecules *(1)* appear in the bloodstream, monocytes *(2)*, a type of white blood cell, transform into macrophages *(3)* that attack the "invaders." Both start to stick to the cells that line the artery wall. As they accumulate, they become foam cells *(4)* and penetrate the artery's inner lining *(5)*, creating fatty streaks. Some of these streaks burst, attracting platelets *(6)* that create clots that trap foam cells and fatty streaks, forming plaque.

2. Oxidized LDL is chemotractic, which just means that it attracts more LDL to the area.

3. As macrophages and LDL continue to build up, the process speeds up. Eventually, your vessel will contain a mass of macrophages. These combine with oxidized LDL and become new types of cells called foam cells. Foam cells are a different type of white blood cell—the kind that is one of the basic components of plaque.

4. These foam cells enter the intima, or inner lining of the arteries, where they start forming fatty streaks. These are exactly what they sound like: streaks of fat growing in your artery walls. Some of these streaks burst, attracting platelets, which are responsible for clotting, to the area. So now you have a clot growing over a mass of foam cells and fatty streaks.

5. The oxidized LDL is toxic to the cells in the arterial wall's intima and starts breaking the vessels' walls down. Your artery becomes less elastic and resilient, aggravating the problems even further.

6. Some researchers even believe that this buildup of cells causes smooth muscle cells to grow in the area as well, which can expand the size of the plaque and, therefore, the risk that it represents by further reducing the diameter of the blood vessel.

This series of plaque formation steps is often prelude to serious heart trouble, including heart attacks. But there is evidence that vitamin E can slow down this domino effect. Here's how.

The chemical structure of vitamin E includes many hydrogen molecules. These molecules effectively offer themselves to the scavenging free radicals—unstable oxygen molecules lacking an electron—before these radicals can link up with the LDL and start plaque formation. The marriage of radicals and hydrogen doesn't produce the dangerous foam cells that enter the lining of your blood vessels. Instead, when two hydrogen molecules unite with a free (oxygen) radical, the result is H_2O, also known as water, also known as good for your body.

Vitamin E can enter your arterial walls on its own. But because it's fat-soluble, it can also attach itself directly to LDL molecules. So your LDL molecules can actually arm themselves with the hydrogen molecules that thwart the plaque-building process by preventing the LDL–free radical merger. Either way, vitamin E can roam freely through your circulatory system, scavenging for rogue free radicals before they can do their damage.

There is evidence for some other mechanisms of vitamin E plaque prevention and heart protection.

■ *Many scientists believe that vitamin E affects the ability of platelets to clump together, or aggregate. In other words, it slows down the blood-clotting process by making platelets less sticky. Since blood clots are an integral component of plaque, this slows down plaque formation.*

■ *There is some evidence that vitamin E can slow down smooth muscle overgrowth in the coronary artery. This is critically important because that overgrowth is a major component of blockages of the vessels that nourish the heart.*

Impressive Clinical Evidence

Since the early 1990s, many studies from around the world have shown that vitamin E acts against heart disease by reducing free radical activity. After the early studies on piglets and rodents in the 1980s, researchers from various institutions followed up with persuasive studies with humans.

They gave half the participants high doses of vitamin E and the other half a placebo. After a couple of weeks, they took blood from both groups and bombarded the blood samples in the test tubes with oxygen. The results showed that there was less oxidation of the LDLs among the people who had taken the vitamin E supplements. Less oxidation, as you'll recall from our discussion in chapter 5, means less free radical damage.

Fred Gey, M.D., a researcher based in Basel, Switzerland, con-

A Couple of Cautions

In general, even at high doses, vitamin E is perfectly safe. Some people, when they start supplementing, may experience a slight case of gastric upset, which subsides in a few days. There is, however, one important warning to keep in mind.

If you're taking a prescription blood thinner or an anti-clotting drug, including warfarin, also marketed as coumidin, be wary of taking vitamin E supplements. Because vitamin E has an anti-clotting effect, the two substances in combination could result in excessive bleeding, even hemorrhage. Vitamin E can sometimes interfere with the absorption and action of vitamin K, which is involved in blood coagulation. If you've had a stroke or bleeding problems, be sure to consult your doctor before taking vitamin E supplements.

Your doctor is the best source of information on good and bad supplement and drug combinations. Never start taking a supplement without consulting him or her.

ducted an important study of vitamin E. Dr. Gey launched one of the world's first international studies of the effect of vitamins on heart health. He compared vitamin E levels in the blood of randomly selected men who lived in several different areas of Europe. His study included men from North Karelia in Finland; Edinborough, Scotland (regions that have relatively high rates of coronary disease); Belfast, Northern Ireland (where there is a medium rate of coronary disease); Thun, Switzerland; and Capri, Italy (where the rate of disease is relatively low).

Gey's results, published in *The American Journal of Clinical Nutrition* in 1987, demonstrated that the people in countries with higher rates of heart disease generally had less vitamin E in their blood. In a subsequent study, Gey found that the higher the level of vitamin E in people's blood, the less likely they were to die of heart disease.

Though these results were interesting, they were by no means definitive. Even Dr. Gey himself raised important questions about his findings. What if the diets or lifestyles of the heart-healthier countries contained another unmeasured protective ingredient in addition to, or even instead of, vitamin E? For this kind of cross-cultural study, it was just very difficult to isolate variables, to take into account all of the factors that might contribute to heart health. It wasn't until 1993 that another large study about vitamin E and its cardiac benefits appeared.

Two careful studies, independently conducted, provided historic results. One was led by prominent researchers Meir Stampfer, M.D., Dr.PH, professor of epidemiology and nutrition at Harvard School of Public Health; the other by Eric Rimm, D.Sc., assistant professor of nutrition and epidemiology at the Harvard School of Public Health. As part of a major health study published in 1993, Dr. Rimm and his team monitored about 40,000 male physicians between the ages of 45 and 70. The results, published in the *New England Journal of Medicine*, were impressive. They showed that men who took 100 IU or more of vitamin E daily for at least 2 years enjoyed almost a 40 percent reduction in risk of heart disease.

The Rimm results were impressive because the study included a large sample of people who were studied over years and because the researchers accounted for other factors that might have affected their likelihood of getting coronary heart disease: obesity, fat intake, and other vitamins or nutrients. They found that only vitamin E had this protective effect. And it protected smokers and nonsmokers alike.

How much vitamin E did people need to enjoy this protective effect? In Dr. Rimm's study, the people who took as little as 100 IU enjoyed as much protection against heart disease as those who took 1,000 IU of vitamin E. Approximately 40 percent of them reduced their risk of heart disease. As long as their daily vitamin E dose exceeded 100 IU, they enjoyed this beneficial effect.

Dr. Stampfer's study had similar good news for women. Since 1976, he has been one of the physicians running the Nurses' Health Study at Harvard. This study has followed more than 85,000 women who were between ages 34 and 59 when the study began. On the question of vitamin E as a cardiovascular protective agent, Dr. Stampfer reported the same protective benefit for women, but it required twice the amount of vitamin E to achieve that benefit. Women who took more than 200 IU of vitamin E daily for at least 2 years had a 40 percent reduction in coronary risk compared with women taking little or no vitamin E. In other words, women who took high doses of vitamin E demonstrated a significant reduction compared with those who took only low doses.

A Vitamin E Profile

What it is:
A fat-soluble vitamin

What it does:
Neutralizes harmful free oxygen radicals in your blood

Mechanism of protection:
Keeps low-density lipoprotein (LDL, or "bad") cholesterol from forming plaque in your arteries

Where you can buy it:
Pharmacies, health food stores, and supermarkets

What to look for on the label:
Vitamin E or D-alpha-tocopherol or DL-alpha-tocopherol

Who it's for:
Adults over age 30

How much to take:
400 IU daily if you're healthy, 800 IU if you already have heart disease; it is particularly important to consult your doctor if you take vitamin E in the latter case

Like Dr. Rimm's study of men, the Nurses' Health Study at Harvard also took into account other variables that might have influenced the subjects' heart health, including age, dietary differences, and exercise habits.

Dr. Stampfer and Dr. Rimm are even encouraged by their one potentially discouraging finding: Their studies demonstrated that you have to take vitamin E for at least 2 years before it shows a protective effect on your heart.

They believe that this finding endorses vitamin E because it fits the biology of plaque formation. Atherosclerosis is a long process. And if vitamin E does what we medical experts think it does, it's most effective at the early stages of plaque development. So, it makes sense that it would take a while before vitamin E's early antioxidant assistance would show up. It's not that it takes 2 years for vitamin E to start working; it starts working immediately. But the results are not measurable for a little while. Or, as Dr. Rimm put it, "the finding that the apparent benefit of vitamin E supplements was stronger with longer-term use is further evidence of a specific effect."

Other clinical studies since the Stampfer and Rimm studies support their findings. One study, published in the *New England Journal of Medicine* in 1994, looked at the effect of vitamin E (as well as beta-carotene) on almost 30,000 male smokers in Finland. After 5 to 7 years, the men taking even small supplements of vitamin E—50 IU—had lower rates of heart disease. The study also showed that those people taking vitamin E who had already had heart attacks at the outset of the study had fewer nonfatal heart attacks than those not taking vitamin E. By way of explaining nonfatal heart attacks, the dose of vitamin E in this study was low compared with other studies that report beneficial cardiac protective effects. This could, in part, explain the lack of an effect on fatal heart attacks.

Though the details of the evidence vary from study to study, the research into vitamin E and cardiac health has remarkable overall consistency. Whether the studies are cross-cultural, strictly observational, or clinical trials testing the effects of many supplements, the results have been the same: Vitamin E can lower your risk of heart disease.

Here's how Dr. Rimm summarizes the wide-ranging good news: "It looks like vitamin E protects smokers, nonsmokers, people who don't exercise, and those who do. Within all the statistical power that we brought to our studies, it looks like vitamin E lowers the risk of coronary disease across the board."

Vitamin E and the Second Heart Attack

If you've already had a heart attack, vitamin E supplements may help protect you from a second one.

The evidence is in a study, called the Cambridge Heart Antioxidant Study, or CHAOS, conducted in England by a team of researchers led by Nigel G. Stephens, M.D., and published in *The Lancet* in 1996.

The CHAOS researchers wanted to find out whether vitamin E could reduce the risks of heart attack or death in people who already had heart disease. They randomly assigned 2,000 people who had confirmed cases of coronary disease to take either vitamin E supplements (in doses ranging from 400 to 800 IU) or a placebo.

A year or so later, in the vitamin E group, 14 people had had nonfatal heart attacks, compared with 41 people who took the placebo. People taking the vitamin E for a year or more were 77 percent less likely to suffer nonfatal heart attacks. And overall, vitamin E reduced the risk of having a nonfatal heart attack or dying of heart disease by 47 percent. According to the CHAOS results, vitamin E did not show any effect on the risk of dying of heart disease. But anything that reduces the risk of having a heart attack is clearly worth taking.

Furthermore, think back to the findings of Dr. Rimm and Dr. Stampfer. They found that it takes up to 2 years for vitamin E to have a measurable effect. Most of the people who died during the CHAOS study did so during the early part of the follow-up period.

The researchers concluded that daily doses of vitamin E (ranging from 400 to 800 IU) could help prevent nonfatal heart attacks while other studies report a preventive effect for both fatal and nonfatal heart attacks. In medicine, particularly in studies with large numbers of patients, it is not uncommon to have mixed results. This could be one reason why there are differences reported about nonfatal versus fatal heart attacks.

Other studies have since corroborated these results. One team, for instance, assessed the progression of plaque in coronary arteries of 162 nonsmoking men ages 40 to 59. The plaque of those who took at least 100 IU of vitamin E daily grew much more slowly than the plaque of the non–vitamin takers. Researchers looking at the carotid arteries (the big ones in the neck leading to the brain) in the same group of men discovered fewer signs of atherosclerosis in those blood vessels as well.

In order to reduce your chances of having a first or second heart attack, it is best to start taking vitamin E at age 30.

Why Supplementation Is Important

Despite the benefits of vitamin E, many people don't even consume the Recommended Dietary Allowance (RDA) of 30 IU, not to mention the 400 IU or more that research suggests. Even Americans who eat well receive only about 30 IU from their diets. Why are so many people walking around deprived of the bare minimum of vitamin E? Because it's very difficult to get all the vitamin E your body can use from food.

To begin with, some of the foods that have the highest concentration of vitamin E—including peanut butter, corn oil, avocados, and nuts—are also high in fat, so the low-fat revolution has led us to cut back on them. But even if we weren't cutting back on these foods, it would still be tough to get enough vitamin E from them. Just as an example, here's how much you'd have to eat of each one of these foods to get 400 IU of vitamin E.

- *6 cups of corn oil*
- *10 cups of peanut butter*
- *100 cups of spinach*
- *48 cups of wheat germ*

Doesn't sound too appealing, does it? Beyond the mere volume problem, much of the vitamin E in our foods is gone long before it ever gets anywhere near our blood vessels. Packaging and processing destroy vitamin E. Milling grain to convert whole wheat to white flour, for example, removes 80 percent of the grain's vitamin E. Canning can deplete almost two-thirds of the vitamin E in some vegetables. Roasting nuts robs them of 80 percent of their vitamin E. Though vitamin E is powerful inside your body, it's as fragile as fine china outside it. Oxygen, heat, light, and even freezing all destroy it.

Supplements are the only practical way to get maximum benefit from vitamin E if you are aiming for 400 IU daily or higher.

The Vitamin E Plan

Even Americans who eat well take in only about 30 IU of vitamin E from their diets. And the RDA for vitamin E is even lower—12 to 15 IU daily, depending on your age and gender. This may be enough to stave off certain deficiency diseases. But it's far too low to reap the extra cardiac benefits of high amounts of vitamin E.

The best way you can protect your heart is through supplementation beginning at age 30. Though clinical studies report that the dose of this substance for the cardiac benefits range from 100 to 1,000 IU, I would recommend the following:

Aim for 400 IU if you're well, 800 IU if you have coronary artery disease. In Dr. Rimm's study, the people who took as little as 100 IU of vitamin E enjoyed as much protection against heart disease as those who took 1,000 IU. But it's best to go for higher doses in order to ensure that you are taking enough. The benefit of 400 IU daily or even 800 IU is accepted by many cardiologists and other physician-experts.

Synthetic will suffice. Vitamin E is available in natural or synthetic formulations. Natural vitamin E is more active in your body than synthetic E, but the difference is taken into account in the packaging measure, the international unit. That means that 100 IU of synthetic E is as potent as 100 IU of natural E.

Which Is More Dangerous: High Cholesterol or Low Vitamin E?

The importance of keeping our cholesterol levels down has become a kind of national health chorus. And even though most people who have heart trouble don't have high cholesterol, it's nonetheless clear that low cholesterol is better for your health than high cholesterol. But there is some evidence to suggest that low levels of vitamin E may actually be a better predictor of heart disease than high cholesterol.

One study conducted among men in 17 western European countries pointed out that high blood cholesterol was predictive of heart disease only 29 percent of the time, and high blood pressure was predictive 25 percent of the time. But low blood levels of vitamin E predicted a heart attack almost 70 percent of the time.

It's only one study. But keep in mind that although vitamin E supplements won't lower the level of the cholesterol in your system, they will lower the threat that cholesterol represents. By keeping the LDLs in your system from combining with free radicals—those unstable molecules roaming in search of electrons—and starting plaque formation, vitamin E has the net effect of making cholesterol less dangerous to the well-being of your blood vessels.

Most of the studies to which I've referred throughout this chapter used synthetic vitamin E. Since it's less expensive, I recommend using it, though there is nothing wrong with taking natural vitamin E. To know which kind of vitamin E your supplement has, read the list of ingredients. Natural E is a D-alpha-tocopherol; synthetic E is DL-alpha-tocopherol. Some scientists believe that gamma-tocopherol is a better form of vitamin E, but this issue is still controversial.

Store them right. Vitamin E capsules should be stored in a cool, dark place. When exposed to air, heat, and light, the capsules can lose their potency.

Summing Up E Supplements

Vitamin E can protect many of us. Even if you're perfectly healthy, taking 400 international units daily is a wise disease-prevention habit. It is particularly important for people who either have heart problems already or have risk factors for heart disease. I strongly recommend these supplements for people with high cholesterol levels, with a strong family history of heart disease, with coronary artery disease, with myocardial ischemia or angina, and for people who have had a heart attack or are at high risk for a stroke.

Always consult your doctor before starting a supplement program. Vitamin E supplementation is extremely safe, unless you are on blood-thinning or anti-clotting medication.

CHAPTER NINE

The B-Vitamin Shield

Like cholesterol, homocysteine is a crucial ingredient for our health. It's an amino acid and has an important role in protein synthesis and many metabolic processes. Homocysteine plays a part in a sequence of biochemical conversions. It converts another amino acid, methionine—found in red meat, milk, and other foods—into a substance called cystathionine, which in turns produces a vital building-block protein called cysteine.

But beware of too much of a good thing. When we have too much homocysteine, it can turn from a vital substance into a health danger.

Normally, the homocysteine in your blood is either reprocessed—used over and over again as part of this protein metabolism cycle—or excreted. But sometimes, there's a problem, and high levels of homocysteine can start building up in your blood. Since the early 1990s, clinical studies have reported that abnormally high levels of this substance are a risk factor for coronary artery disease and heart attacks.

The American Medical Association now considers high homocysteine levels in your blood to be an independent risk factor for heart disease. But while everyone—researchers, physicians, and drug

126

companies—was figuring out ways to beat high cholesterol, the issue of homocysteine was essentially overlooked.

Even if you have normal cholesterol levels, even if you eat a high-fiber, low-fat diet, even if you exercise regularly, you may still have elevated levels of homocysteine. Neither a low-fat dietary regime or rigorous exercise can control your homocysteine level. But there is a nutraceutical approach to this problem.

The proper amounts of a trio of B vitamins can keep your homocysteine level in check. The B vitamins—folic acid, also known as folate, vitamin B_6, and vitamin B_{12}—play an essential role in the biochemical reactions that turn homocysteine into methionine. (The evidence is not so strong regarding vitamin B_6.) They are also critical to the process that turns excess homocysteine into substances that can be excreted by our bodies. In a way, the B vitamins are ecologists—they control homocysteine by making sure that it's either reprocessed or thrown away.

Before exploring the research that endorses the use of B vitamins to battle homocysteine, let's look at the medical history behind this too-little-known potential threat to our heart health.

A Medical Pioneer and a Delayed Opportunity

We should have been concerned about homocysteine long ago. But unfortunately, back in the late 1960s, the pioneering work of a forward-looking young doctor wasn't given the attention that it deserved.

Kilmer S. McCully, M.D., was a researcher at Harvard Medical School when he became intrigued by the case reports on two youngsters—one 8 years old, the other only 2 months old—who were dying of advanced atherosclerosis. They had been stricken by a rare genetic disease called homocystinuria, an ailment characterized by abnormally high blood levels of homocysteine. Since these children had a disease normally associated with middle, or even old, age, Dr. McCully wondered whether there might be a connection between high blood levels of homocysteine and cardio-

Nutraceutical Tandems: Folate and Its Partners

Remember the principle of nutraceutical synergy that I described in chapter 4? This is the idea that the combinations of nutraceuticals can be especially effective against coronary artery and heart disease. Here are two excellent illustrations.

The study by Eric Rimm, D.Sc., assistant professor of nutrition and epidemiology at the Harvard School of Public Health, and his group that showed folate to be an effective cardiovascular nutraceutical also showed that the women who had the highest intake of vitamin B_6 were 30 percent less likely to get coronary artery disease than the women who had the lowest intake of B_6. Interestingly, however, the study found that the women who had the highest intake of both folate and vitamin B_6 had the greatest protection of all: a 45 percent reduction in risk compared to those with low intakes of both vitamins. The study concluded that eating about twice the Recommended Dietary Allowance (RDA) of folate and B_6 could significantly reduce a woman's risk of heart disease.

Dr. Rimm also found that the nutraceutical alcohol added to folates could offer additional protection. The high-folate women who also had one or more drinks a day had a greater reduction of the number of heart attacks than the other groups. Combining high folate with alcohol was reported to cut the risk by 80 percent, about twice as much as folate or alcohol alone.

vascular disease in general. Like a lot of medical research, Dr. McCully's began with animal studies. He injected rabbits with homocysteine and found that within a matter of weeks, they developed atherosclerosis. By 1969, Dr. McCully was ready to go public with his homocysteine studies. He published a paper in the *American Journal of Pathology* postulating that elevated homocysteine levels could be a major factor responsible for plaque buildup leading to cardiovascular disease. Dr. McCully also suggested that some or all of the B-complex vitamins could bring homocysteine levels down to normal.

At the time, the medical establishment was enamored with cholesterol as a risk factor for heart disease, and Dr. McCully's results were given little credence. He was forced to leave Harvard. He continued his research on homocysteine and the B vitamins at the Department of Veterans Affairs Medical Center in Providence, Rhode Island. It's a tragedy that the medical establishment didn't give Dr. McCully's research more attention and did not appreciate what he tried to tell us about the importance of controlling homocysteine.

A New Heart Disease Suspect at Last

In terms of public health, the question of homocysteine got very little attention for more than 2 decades, until 1992, when Meir Stampfer, M.D., Dr.PH, professor of epidemiology and nutrition at Harvard School of Public Health, and his colleagues published the results of a 10-year-long research project called the Physicians' Health Study. Dr. Stampfer and his colleagues had been taking blood samples from and monitoring the diet and health of almost 15,000 male doctors between the ages of 40 and 84. This study had achieved some national recognition because, a few year earlier, it had determined that taking aspirin resulted in a 44 percent reduction in heart attacks.

But the Stampfer team was also interested in homocysteine levels. Their findings supported Dr. McCully's original observations from the 1960s. Many of the men who had heart attacks had considerably higher levels of homocysteine in their blood than those who stayed healthy. And, in a way even more significant, those with the very highest levels of homocysteine were more than three times more likely to have a heart attack.

The researchers were careful to be sure that there was no association between these high homocysteine levels and the presence or absence of other commonly known risk factors for heart disease, such as high blood pressure, diabetes, or angina. In other words, the

If You Take Folate Supplements, Take B₁₂ Too

The clinical evidence in support of folate supplements is, in my opinion, persuasive. At this point in time, I would recommend 400 micrograms of folate a day. And if you take folate supplements, it's especially important that you take B_{12} supplements as well.

Why? Because a high level of folate can do two things: (1) It can offer effective protection for your arteries, and (2) it can mask a deficiency of B_{12}.

People with pernicious anemia or people taking an anticonvulsant medication should consult with their physicians. High intake of folic acids can mask the signs of pernicious anemia and might interfere with the effectiveness of anticonvulsants.

study demonstrated that a high homocysteine level alone is a risk factor for heart disease.

This study was among the first after Dr. McCully's to demonstrate the homocysteine–heart health connection, and it precipitated a wave of research into homocysteine as a cardiovascular risk factor. Here are just a few of the studies that have verified the link.

■ *A 1995 study of almost 22,000 patients in Norway tried to quantify the high homocysteine risk. It found that, for both men and women, the risk of developing coronary artery disease was statistically higher with every 4-microgram increase in homocysteine level.*

■ *Also in 1995, researcher Carol J. Boushey, R.D., Ph.D., of the University of Washington in Seattle, and others published a meta-analysis of 38 studies on homocysteine in the* Journal of the American Medical Association. *It was an analysis of every major reputable study on the subject done up until that time. The studies clearly showed that the higher the level of homocysteine, the more likely people were to have cardiovascular disease. In another attempt to quantify the risk, the researchers estimated that each 5-microgram increase in blood homocysteine was associated with a 60 percent (for men) and 80 percent (for women) increase in risk of developing heart disease (coronary artery disease).*

■ *An international study of men in 13 different countries, conducted by the World Health Organization and published in* The Lancet *in 1997, found a strong correlation between high homocysteine levels in healthy men between ages 40 and 49 and a higher death rate from cardiovascular disease.*

■ *A team headed by researcher Nicholas Wald, D.Sc., Fellow of the Royal College of Physicians, of the Department of Environmental and Preventative Medicine in London, did an interesting historical study that was published in the journal* Archives of Internal Medicine *in 1998. They accessed the records of more than 20,000 healthy men who had been treated at a medical center in London between 1975 and 1982 as part of an earlier study. They compared the homocysteine levels of the 229 men who eventually died of heart disease with 1,126 healthy men. They found significantly high homocysteine levels among the men who got heart disease. Their results agreed with Dr. Stampfer's study that the risk of heart disease was three times greater for people with the highest levels of homocysteine.*

There have also been revealing studies done of homocysteine levels in people whose cardiovascular systems may already be compromised.

■ *A study published in the* New England Journal of Medicine *in 1996 explored a connection between homocysteine levels in patients with lupus erythematosus, commonly known as lupus, and their risk of having a stroke. The researchers chose to study patients with lupus because they are particularly vulnerable to stroke. Their study found that high levels of homocysteine were associated with increased clot formation as well as a higher incidence of stroke.*

■ *Another study conducted by Marion Hofman, M.D., of the department of medicine at the University of Heidelberg in Germany, published in* Diabetes Care *in 1997, looked at the link between high levels of homocysteine and plaque buildup in the small arteries of 75 people with diabetes. People with diabetes are at a higher risk of cardiac disease than the general population. They tend to develop endothelial dysfunction, which is plaque buildup in the inner linings of their arteries. The researchers found that the people with diabetes had higher homocysteine levels than healthy control subjects. And higher homocysteine levels were linked with higher levels of endothelial dysfunction.*

■ *Perhaps most persuasive of all is a study done by Ottar Nygard, M.D., of the department of heart disease at Haukeland University Hospital in Norway and published in 1997 in the* New England Journal of Medicine. *Dr. Nygard's group measured the homocysteine levels of almost 600 patients who already had coronary artery disease. They found a strong correlation between the subjects' homocysteine readings and the likelihood that the heart disease would kill them. The higher the levels of homocysteine in their blood, the more likely they were to die. Within 4 years, only 4 percent of the patients with low homocysteine died, but 25 percent of those with high readings fell victim to the disease.*

■ *A more recent study, the Rotterdam Study, was conducted with 7,983 patients in the Netherlands. The purpose was to evaluate relationships between the level of homocysteine and stroke in the elderly population. The conclusion of the clinical research is that there is indeed an association: The higher the level, the greater the cardiovascular risk.*

There is also evidence that homocysteine could be particularly dangerous to postmenopausal women. In a study published in 1999 in the *Journal of the American Medical Association*, Paul Ridker, M.D., of the Division of Cardiovascular Diseases and Preventative Medicine at Brigham and Women's Hospital in Boston, analyzed 29,000 postmenopausal women who had been participants in the

Women's Health Study since 1993. His research team found that women with the highest levels of homocysteine were twice as likely to die of cardiovascular disease as women who had the lowest levels.

Though by now clinical studies have clearly shown that high homocysteine is somehow linked to heart disease, it's still far from clear exactly how homocysteine undermines our cardiovascular health.

Leading Theories on Homocysteine's Effects

Too much homocysteine causes damage to the inside walls of the arteries, which leads to plaque buildup. The precise mechanism by which this happens is still unclear. In fact, homocysteine may damage the arteries in several different ways. Here are a few of the leading theories.

■ *Too much homocysteine may create free radicals, which I mentioned in chapter 8 in connection with vitamin E's role as an antioxidant. These free radicals bind with low-density lipoproteins (LDLs) to begin the process of plaque formation.*

■ *Homocysteine may make arteries less resilient by breaking down the tissues on arterial walls. This makes the vessels less capable of constricting and dilating normally.*

■ *Excessive homocysteine may encourage the smooth muscle cells in arterial walls to multiply. This, too, can narrow the vessels.*

■ *Homocysteine may increase blood coagulation or affect the action of thrombin (one of the basic clotting components). This can cause blood clots to form around already existing plaques.*

Beyond the question of how homocysteine does its damage is the still-open question of why homocysteine levels get elevated in the first place.

Fortunately, we do know what to do about elevated levels of

homocysteine. Nutraceutical supplements of B vitamins—folic acid, B_6, and B_{12}—can slow down the accumulation of homocysteine.

Folic Acid: The Enemy of Homocysteine

Folic acid has lots of names and lots of functions in the body. Its official name is pteroylglutamic acid, though it's often referred to as folate when it's in food. The name comes from the Latin word *folium*, meaning "leaf" or "foliage." It was so named because it was first found, back in 1941, in spinach.

Folic acid is responsible for several life-sustaining functions. It plays a role in the metabolism of protein and in the formation of blood cells. Folic acid is also crucial in the development and repair of both DNA and RNA, the components of our genes and chromosomes. That's why pregnant women often take supplements of folic acid to prevent neural tube birth defects such as spina bifida.

Literally dozens of studies from around the world, including tens of thousands of subjects, have confirmed that folic acid fights heart disease by breaking down homocysteine so that it can be cleared from our systems. "I think there's tremendously strong evidence that if you give people folate, their homocysteine levels go down," said Dr. Stampfer in a personal interview. "You can even put people on different doses of folate, and it has an effect. If someone takes an average of 500 micrograms of folates daily, their homocysteine levels will go down. And if they take a higher dose, their homocysteine goes down even more."

In 1985, a Finnish researcher, Lars Brattstrom, of the department of medicine at the County Hospital in Kalmar, Sweden, reported that giving healthy people folic acid reduced their homocysteine levels by an average of 30 percent. Brattstrom reported that folic acid seemed to reduce all but low homocysteine levels.

Howard Morrison, Ph.D., and his colleagues at the Cancer Bureau in Ottawa, Canada, did a study that demonstrated the cardio-

Foods High in Folate

In response to the growing body of evidence that folic acid is essential for health, the FDA began a folate fortification program in 1998, requiring that folate be added to pasta, breads, enriched flours, rice, and all other grain products. Even so, it's still very difficult to get enough folate from your diet. The following chart will give you a good idea of how much you'd need to eat to meet the 400 micrograms that I've recommended for heart health.

Food	Amount	Folate (mcg)
Lentils	1 cup	358
Chickpeas	1 cup	282
Lima beans	1 cup	273
Black beans	1 cup	256
Kidney beans	1 cup	229
Beef liver	3.5 oz	220
Great northern beans	1 cup	213
Asparagus	6 spears	131
Spinach	½ cup	131
Wheat germ	¼ cup	102
Chicory greens	½ cup	99
Soybeans	1 cup	93
Brussels sprouts	½ cup	80
Sunflower seeds	1 oz	67
Peanuts	1 oz	41
Corn	½ cup	40
Chinese cabbage	½ cup	35
Broccoli	½ cup	31
Cantaloupe	1 cup	27
Strawberries	1 cup	26
Sweet potato	1	26
Oatmeal	½ cup	20
Oranges	1	5

protective activity of folate. Dr. Morrison and his colleagues assessed more than 5,000 men and women between the ages of 35 and 79 who had no personal medical history of heart disease. He measured their folate levels as well as their heart disease risk factors. Thirteen years later, he assessed their health status.

Dr. Morrison found that the people with the lowest folate levels were statistically most likely to get coronary heart disease. Though it was difficult to separate out other cardiac risk factors, including hypertension (high blood pressure) and high cholesterol, one fact stood out: The higher the folate level, the less prone to coronary heart disease these thousands of men and women were. When it came to heart disease fatalities, the results were particularly impressive. The people with the lowest levels of folate in their blood were 69 percent more likely to die of a heart attack than those with the highest levels.

Can Diet Supply Sufficient Folic Acid?

There are many good food sources of folic acid. Theoretically, it's possible to get the amounts that offer heart protection benefits from your diet. You would have to eat five to nine servings of fruits and vegetables daily, plus some folate-fortified bread and cereal.

In reality, the average American diet is deficient in folic acid. According to a study published in the *American Journal of Clinical Nutrition*, 59 percent of middle-aged men are deficient in folic acid. This deficiency is defined by the Recommended Dietary Allowance, which is not enough to sufficiently prevent atherosclerosis.

According to the 1995 University of Washington meta-analysis conducted by Dr. Boushey in Seattle, almost 90 percent of our population consumes less than the minimum 400 micrograms of folate that you need every day to keep your homocysteine levels down. Even though many breads and flours are now fortified with

Good Food Sources of Vitamin B₁₂

You want to take 500 to 1,000 micrograms of B_{12} daily. If you really like to eat liver and organ meats, you might actually be able to pull that off, assuming that your intestines break down and absorb all the B_{12} that you eat. This chart gives you a good idea of why supplements are so important.

Food	Amount	B₁₂ (mcg)
Clams	3 oz	84
Bluefish	3 oz	5.29
Lamb	3.5 oz	2.6
Milk	8 oz	1
Eggs	1 large	0.56
Anchovies	5	0.18

folate, average consumption of many of them will raise your folate intake by only 120 micrograms or less.

A 1998 study by Michael Malinow, M.D., with the division of pathobiology and immunology and the division of reproductive sciences at Oregon Regional Primate Research Center, and others focused on three groups of people. The first group had cereal fortified with 125 micrograms of folate, which only reduced the amount of homocysteine in people's blood by about 3.7 percent. However, when people regularly had cereal containing higher levels of folate fortification (499 and 665 micrograms, respectively, for the other two groups), homocysteine in their blood decreased by 11 percent and 14 percent, respectively. The researchers suggested that folic acid fortification at levels higher than recommended by the FDA made a lot of sense.

Perhaps the most persuasive of all the studies about the homocysteine-inhibiting ability of folates were the findings of Eric

Rimm, D.Sc., assistant professor of nutrition and epidemiology at the Harvard School of Public Health, and his team. They provided clinical evidence that folate and vitamin B$_6$ could prevent heart disease among women.

Dr. Rimm and his group at Harvard have been tracking the health of more than 80,000 American women for many years as part of a diet and health study known as the Nurses' Health Study. Although all the women were healthy at the outset of the study, over its course, 658 had nonfatal heart attacks and 281 had heart attacks that killed them. When the women were assessed over the years, the researchers found that:

- *The women who consumed the most folate had about a 30 percent reduction in risk of coronary disease compared to those with the lowest intake of folate.*
- *The more folate the women took, the lower their risk of coronary artery disease.*
- *Every 100-microgram increase in folate consumption was associated with 6 percent less homocysteine and a 5.8 percent lower risk of heart disease.*
- *The lowest risk for heart disease was among women who took more than 400 micrograms daily.*

Vitamin B$_{12}$ Can Slow Down Homocysteine Buildup

Back in the 1920s, researchers at Harvard Medical School made an interesting discovery. They found that people with pernicious anemia, a rare and sometimes fatal blood disorder, could survive as long as they ate ⅔ of a pound of raw liver daily. But it took 20 years before anybody figured out why: Liver is rich in vitamin B$_{12}$, which helped the anemia patients fight the disease.

How's Your Homocysteine?

The normal range of homocysteine in blood is less than 6 to 9 micrograms per liter. If the amount in your own blood is higher than 15 micrograms per liter, you could have hyperhomocystinemia, dangerous excess of homocysteine in your blood, which should be treated by a doctor. Ask your doctor about laboratory tests for blood and urine now available to measure your homocysteine level.

Vitamin B_{12}, also called cobalamin, has the most complex chemical structure of all the vitamins. It plays a central role in many biological functions, including the formation of red blood cells and the production of myelin, the fatty sheath that surrounds nerve fibers. It can also help fight coronary artery disease by lowering homocysteine levels. Though researchers haven't yet figured out the mechanism through which it works, many studies strongly suggest that it does indeed lower homocysteine.

Other research supports this role of vitamin B_{12}. Dr. Robert Clarke and an international group of investigators based in Oxford University in England analyzed 12 clinical studies that had assessed the effects of folic acid supplements—with or without vitamins B_6 and B_{12}—on blood homocysteine concentration. The results, published in 1998 in the *British Medical Journal*, made a compelling case for B_{12} as a homocysteine controller.

Like the other studies of folate, Dr. Clarke's study found that folate lowered homocysteine. Interestingly, however, they also found that adding vitamin B_{12} to the B-vitamin mix produced an additional drop in homocysteine levels. In fact, the results suggest that a daily dose of at least 0.5 milligrams of folic acid and about 0.5 milligrams daily of vitamin B_{12} should reduce blood homocysteine by about a quarter to a third.

How can you tell if you're deficient in B_{12}? If you're extremely deficient, you'll get very tired. Too little B_{12} slows down your production of oxygen-bearing red blood cells, and too little oxygen means not much energy. Since a severe B_{12} shortage limits your body's ability to repair the myelin that protects your nerves, you may experience nerve-related symptoms, including memory loss, confusion, balance problems, or tingling of the hands and feet.

Clinical B_{12} deficiency is plenty common. An estimated 800,000 Americans have it, and in some cases, it can be quite serious. But for purposes of this discussion, the bigger issue is subclinical B_{12} deficiency, a shortage of vitamin B_{12} that has no detectable symptoms. Experts, including Dr. Stampfer, who has done some of the large population studies, believe that the prevalence of people who should have higher levels of B_{12} is quite high. A study published in the *American Journal of Clinical Nutrition* in 1993 reported that 25 percent of middle-aged men are deficient in B_{12}.

In general, B_{12} deficiency gets more common as we get older. As we age, our stomachs tend to produce less and less of the gastric acid required to liberate B_{12} from food. So, even though we may consume the same amount of B_{12}, functionally, we're short of this key nutrient.

But let me reiterate one of the underlying nutraceutical principles. Our goal mustn't be merely to consume the proper diets in order to survive but, rather, to get the additional amounts, to give ourselves as much nutraceutical protection as possible. Taking B_{12} supplements along with folic acid is a good idea.

B_{12} is available in many foods. Unfortunately, many of them are foods that are out of vogue in our low-fat, anti–red meat age, such as meats, milk, cheese, and eggs. Unlike many other vitamins, B_{12} can't be synthesized by plants, so you won't find it in fruits or vegetables.

Vitamin B_6: The Mystery Guest in the Elixir

Vitamin B_6 is, like most nutrients, tremendously versatile. It helps more than 60 different enzymes do their jobs. Vitamin B_6 is also essential for the formation of blood proteins, for inhibiting platelet aggregation, and for regulating our cells' electrolyte balance. It also plays a role in protein metabolism.

Of the three B vitamins in the Cardiac Elixir, B_6 is the mystery guest. It protects you from heart disease in a different way than folate and B_{12}, both of which work by lowering your homocysteine level. Researchers don't know exactly how B_6 does its prophylactic work. It may be that it, too, lowers homocysteine, but the biochemistry of homocysteine has not yet been fully decoded, and scientists are still groping for an explanation.

As Dr. Rimm put it in a recent interview, "Homocysteine may be more than just a single entity. It may be that the homocysteine you have at fasting levels may be important, and the homocysteine that you might have after a high-protein meal may be different and yet just as important a risk factor."

Dr. Rimm's Nurses' Health Study found that the women who had the highest levels of B_6 had a 30 percent lower risk of heart disease than the women who had the lowest levels.

Another major research project, the European Concerted Action Project, explored the links between ischemic heart disease and dietary supplements at 19 different centers in nine different countries. Its results confirmed not only that high homocysteine put people at special risk but also that all three B vitamins offered heart protection. It also showed that those patients with higher levels of B_6 had greater protection from ischemic heart disease.

Impressive evidence for the effectiveness of vitamin B_6 comes from the Atherosclerosis Risk in Communities Study, published by Aaron R. Folsom, M.D., and others in *Circulation*. Dr. Folsom and his team at the University of Minnesota studied almost 16,000 men and women ages 45 to 64 living in four different communities. His researchers found a correlation between the presence of all three B vitamins and levels of homocysteine. As to B_6, the study showed that heart disease was 70 percent lower among people who had the highest levels of vitamin B_6 in their blood at the start of the study than it was in people who had the lowest.

Good Food Sources of Uitamin B₆

Four tiny milligrams may not sound like a lot. But most foods don't have anywhere close to that amount. Here's a list of foods that are high in B₆. As you can see, you'll have a hard time getting the recommended levels—400 to 500 milligrams daily—if you don't take a supplement.

Food	Amount	B₆ (mg)
Chickpeas	1 cup	0.90
Baked potato	1	0.50
Brown rice	1 cup	0.38
Wheat germ	¼ cup	0.38
Lentils	1 cup	0.35
Navy beans	1 cup	0.30
Sunflower seeds	1 oz	0.23
Spinach	½ cup	0.22
Kidney beans	1 cup	0.21
Lima beans	1 cup	0.14

Vitamin B_6 is available in many foods, including chickpeas, lima beans, kidney beans, lentils, spinach, and brown rice. Nonetheless, it's tough to get enough of this vitamin through your diet to lower your homocysteine levels (see "Good Food Sources of Vitamin B_6"). When you also consider how much vitamin B_6 is lost through cooking and the extent to which stress can increase our nutritional requirements, it's clear that we need supplements to give us every health edge.

One study found that 25 percent of middle-aged men suffer from vitamin B_6 deficiencies. A far greater percentage of people aren't technically B_6 deficient, but could benefit from higher levels.

I recommend 400 to 500 milligrams of vitamin B_6 a day.

Medical Certainties and Your Health

There is skepticism in some medical circles about whether lowering your homocysteine level cuts your risk for ischemic heart disease. I understand where some of my peers are coming from. Most of the studies that I've described are so-called epidemiological studies, meaning that they measure large populations and rely upon statistical analyses. Physicians generally prefer evidence from clinical studies, especially double-blind randomized studies, where half the subjects are given the substance to be evaluated, such as pharmaceuticals and nutraceuticals, and half are given a placebo. The American Heart Association, for example, is reluctant to recommend supplementation with the B vitamins until such gold-standard studies—which are now underway in both Europe and the United States—demonstrate that it reduces ischemic coronary artery disease.

I believe that it is wise medicine for doctors to advise certain patients with and without heart

A B-Vitamin Profile

What they are:
Folate, B_6, and B_{12}, three of the complex B vitamins

What they do:
Lower blood levels of an amino acid called homocysteine

Mechanism of protection:
Homocysteine can contribute to the formation of plaque in your arteries; too much homocysteine is a risk factor for both heart attack and stroke

Where you can buy them:
Pharmacies, health food stores, and supermarkets

What to look for on the label:
Check that your multiple vitamin contains all three—folic acid, vitamin B_6, and vitamin B_{12}; you can also buy them separately if you want to customize the amount of each you take

Who they're for:
Adults with and without heart disease; aside from its cardio-protective benefits, folate is essential for pregnant women, as it has been shown to help prevent many neural tube birth defects

How much to take:
You need 400 to 1,000 micrograms of folic acid daily; 400 to 500 milligrams of vitamin B_6 daily; and 500 to 1,000 micrograms of vitamin B_{12} daily

A Trio of Cautions

In some individuals, folic acid has a paradoxical effect. It actually raises the level of the amino acid homocysteine, and too much is a risk factor for coronary artery disease. Just to be certain that you're not one of those rare people, ask your doctor to measure your homocysteine level before you start taking folic acid and then a little while after you've been supplementing.

People with pernicious anemia and people taking anti-convulsant medications should consult with their doctors before taking supplements of folic acid. High levels of folic acid can mask anemia and interfere with the effectiveness of some anti-seizure medications.

Megadoses of vitamin B_6 can be dangerous.

disease to take supplements of the B vitamins. There's too much evidence of the potential beneficial effects of these nutraceuticals to wait it out.

We know that people with elevated homocysteine levels are more likely to have plaque in their arteries. We know that these nutraceuticals, which are inexpensive and relatively nontoxic, lower homocysteine levels. I think it's wise to take protective action even before all the proof is in. Remember, this is how the "lowering your cholesterol" story began.

The medical community and the government initiated a program to lower cholesterol levels with clinical data similar to what we have about homocysteine. Time has borne this decision out. It is not unreasonable to believe that further research will also support the need to lower high levels of homocysteine.

In other words, take your B vitamins. In the quantities that clinical studies support, they are an important part of the insurance policy against high homocysteine, a positive step that you can take that may reduce your risk of ischemic heart disease.

Summing Up B-Vitamin Supplements

I recommend taking B-vitamin supplements from age 35 on. They can be especially important for people with atherosclerosis in general, and for the more specific types of small artery blockage found in people who have diabetes.

As to risk/benefit analysis, these vitamins are reasonably safe at the supplement levels that I recommend (see "A Trio of Cautions," opposite). Folic acid and vitamin B_{12} are acceptably safe even at high doses, though sometimes high levels of folic acid, or folate, can mask a deficiency in B_{12}. So, if you take folate, it's important to take B_{12} as well.

At this point, it is wise to limit your vitamin B_6 dose to 500 milligrams daily. Vitamin B_6 can be risky in high doses, so don't take levels higher than the recommended dose unless your doctor thinks there's a compelling medical reason for it.

CHAPTER TEN

Magnesium: The Multipurpose Mineral

Throughout this book, I have emphasized the fact that there are no miracle cures. Overstated claims for natural substances are very common in the United States, and I have been frequently critical of these excesses. My goal in writing this book is to share information on certain cardiovascular nutraceuticals generated in clinical studies and supported by medical experts. In other words, we are going to stick to the facts.

But, I confess, when it comes to magnesium, I, too, am tempted to make big claims. Magnesium works in multiple ways throughout your body, and magnesium supplements hold much promise. We've only just begun to tap its potential health benefits. Because magnesium either activates or stabilizes more than 300 different enzyme reactions, it keeps almost every cell in your body functioning properly, including the cells in your cardiovascular system. Your heart muscle cells need magnesium for every single contraction, your arteries need magnesium to stay relaxed and open, and your blood

146

Magnesium Profile

What it is:

A mineral found in the blood and in almost every cell of your body

What it does:

Activates more than 300 different enzyme reactions to maintain cells' mineral balance

Mechanism of protection:

In your heart, it helps keep the cells contracting regularly and stabilizes energy production; in your circulatory system, it can keep your arteries from constricting too much and prevent blood clots; magnesium also can help reduce insulin resistance and helps your body metabolize sugar, both of which can reduce cardiovascular risks for people with diabetes

Where you can buy it:

Pharmacies, health food stores, and supermarkets

What to look for on the label:

Magnesium chloride, magnesium oxide, magnesium gluconate, magnesium animo acids, chelate (chelated magnesium), or magnesium carbonate. Some pills contain only one form, others may include two different types in the same pill

Who it's for:

Adults over age 35; people who have coronary artery disease and cardiomyopathy; people with high blood pressure; people with diabetes

Who it's not for:

Anyone with kidney failure; too much magnesium is dangerous in people with renal disease

How much to take:

400 to 450 milligrams daily

itself needs magnesium to clot normally. But unless you've already started supplementing your diet with magnesium, you're probably not getting enough of it.

On top of this, clinical studies report that magnesium, along with chromium, can reduce insulin resistance. These minerals "change the mind" of cells that would otherwise try to keep insulin and its vital blood sugar–regulating properties out. This last property makes both magnesium and chromium supplements essential, in my opinion, for most people with diabetes. While chromium is not part of the Cardiac Elixir for people without diabetes, it should be included as an additional ingredient for those with diabetes. (See "Chromium: Elixir Nutraceutical for Diabetes," on page 158.)

What Magnesium Does in Your Body

About 60 percent of your body's magnesium is found in your bones, 40 percent is in your muscle and soft tissue, and 1 percent is in extracellular fluids such as the blood. It's everywhere because your cells depend on this mineral in a huge variety of ways and for just about every biochemical reaction. In fact, this would probably be a much shorter chapter if it examined what magnesium *doesn't* do.

In general, magnesium regulates the balance of the other three minerals that you need in your body for your health: calcium, potassium, and sodium. Magnesium ensures just the right electric potential in cell membranes, which is what tells the cell to either accept or reject these minerals. On a practical level, magnesium thus affects how your cell pays attention to what's going on. A cell deficient in magnesium has too much calcium in it, and it becomes irritable. "Irritable" cells are more likely to react to stimuli prematurely or even without provocation, meaning that they might contract when they could relax, or fire off when they could take a break. In contrast, a cell replete with magnesium has more potassium than calcium in it and is more capable of a measured, modulated response. It's more stable.

Following are some ways in which magnesium plays a role in the cardiovascular system.

▪ *In the heart, magnesium stabilizes energy production. You've already learned in chapter 7 that carnitine carries fatty acids—your heart's source of energy—into the mitochondria, or "furnaces" of your heart cells. Energy production is possible when one type of molecule, the ATP (adenosine triphosphate) molecule, is converted into another type, called ADP (adenosine diphosphate) molecule. This conversion can only occur in the presence of fatty acids and oxygen. When ATP turns into ADP, it releases the energy that your heart cells need to stay alive. What I haven't told you until now is that magnesium stabilizes this miraculous energy-producing process. It is an essential component of the metabolic process through which your heart cells produce energy.*

■ *Magnesium keeps your heart beating regularly, helping to prevent arrhythmias. Because it's responsible for keeping mineral levels normal, magnesium plays a critical role—along with sodium, potassium, and calcium—in keeping your heart cells pumping regularly. These substances turn each heart muscle cell into a miniature battery, capable of powerful repeated contractions.*

■ *Magnesium keeps blood pressure stable by acting as nature's calcium channel antagonist—that is, it opposes the action of calcium. The more calcium in your cells, the more "irritable" and likely to overreact they are. You need calcium in your heart muscles because it ensures that they contract vigorously and regularly. And you need your arteries to contract in order to move your blood along.*

But sometimes, calcium proves too much of a good thing. Excessive contractility—a tendency for the artery to contract in your heart muscle cells—can lead to arrhythmias, while excessive contraction or constriction in your arteries can lead to high blood pressure. The more calcium inside your cells, the higher your blood pressure. That's where magnesium comes in. It rides to the rescue in your body and pushes calcium out of cells where it's not needed. Essentially, magnesium calms your cells down. In fact, magnesium acts a lot like the whole class of drugs for heart disease that mimic this action, also called calcium channel antagonists. These drugs reduce calcium's ability to make the heart muscle and blood vessels contract. In effect, they help keep your arteries relaxed. With the arteries relaxed, more blood can get to your heart, which means that your heart doesn't have to work as hard. And it's entirely possible that magnesium may actually work well with drugs like these to broaden their activity. The result is increased blood supply to the heart, which gives the heart less work to do. To date, however, magnesium has not yet been sufficiently evaluated in clinical studies to demonstrate these characteristics.

■ *Magnesium keeps blood pressure stable by acting on nature's angiotensin II inhibitors. Your body has a second way of regulating its blood pressure, and magnesium is intrinsically involved in this process as well. Angiotensin II is medical-ese for the natural vasoconstrictor that your kidney produces. The role of angiotensin II is to constrict your arteries to maintain your blood pressure. Angiotensin II can also raise your blood pressure. But what happens in your body when there's too much angiotensin around, forcing your arteries to clamp down? Your body sends in its magnesium, which inhibits the action of the angiotensin II, thus allowing your blood vessels to open up. The pharmaceutical industry has attempted to mimic the natural effects of magnesium through a class of drugs called ACE (angiotensin converting enzyme) inhibitors. Again, magnesium does this naturally, with no side effects.*

■ *Magnesium affects blood clotting. Various research groups have independently discovered that magnesium reduces the ability of platelets to clump together. Platelets less prone to clumping are also less prone to forming plaque or blocking an artery. One of my colleagues, Jerry Nadler, M.D., an international expert and division chief of endocrinology and metabolism at the University of Virginia in Charlottesville, has conducted extensive research on this subject. He has discovered that when people are magnesium-deficient, whether they have diabetes or not, their blood seems to clot more easily. Dr. Nadler has also found that if you give magnesium-deprived patients magnesium, their blood clotting returns to normal. "We've looked at platelet interactions for many years," he says. "Our results have been validated by other groups as well. Magnesium does reduce platelet reactivity, and that can certainly be translated into potential reductions in cardiac disease."*

■ *Magnesium can help reduce the possibility of plaque formation.*
Remember what you learned about the early stages of plaque for-
mation? It all starts when LDLs (low-density lipoproteins, or
"bad" cholesterol), white blood cells, and platelets start congre-
gating together at your blood vessel wall and turn into plaque. It
turns out that magnesium can actually maintain the integrity of
the inner arterial vessel walls, which can stave off the formation of
the plaque in the first place. It may also actively slow down the rate
at which your LDLs can oxidize.

■ *Magnesium can help your body's insulin push sugar into your*
cells. Along with insulin, magnesium helps feed your cells the nour-
ishment they need in the form of glucose. On top of this, magne-
sium may well play a role in helping cells use their insulin to
metabolize glucose. The cells of people with diabetes don't do these
things very well. Exactly how does magnesium perform these func-
tions? Insulin is a hormone released by your pancreas in response
to normal and high blood sugar levels. Its job is to lower your blood
sugar levels to normal. It does this by attaching itself to special in-
sulin receptors present on the surfaces of body cells, then pushing
the sugar, in the form of glucose, into your cells.

Some people are insulin-resistant. Their insulin can't seem to
push the sugar into the cells. And glucose is a vital source of energy
needed by most living tissue. If your body can't use its insulin ef-
fectively, which is what insulin resistance amounts to, a dangerous
cycle begins. Your blood glucose levels stay high, but your cells are
still deprived of it. Your pancreas reacts to the excess of glucose in
your blood by producing more insulin.

The Dangers of Low Levels

For at least a decade, many groups around the world, including
those led by one of the pioneers of American magnesium research,
Burton Altura, Ph.D., of the department of physiology and the
Center for Cardiovascular and Muscle Research at the State Uni-

Sources of Magnesium in Your Diet

You need 400 to 450 milligrams of magnesium daily to insure adequate stores of the body's magnesium levels. Here's a list of high-magnesium food sources. Think about how frequently you usually eat these foods and how much of them you need to eat every day, and you'll see why just about anyone would have trouble meeting this goal without supplementing.

Magnesium content given here is per 3.5-ounce (100-gram) serving.

Food	Magnesium (mg)
Kelp	760
Wheat bran	490
Wheat germ	336
Almonds	270
Cashews	267
Buckwheat	229
Brazil nuts	225
Filberts	184
Peanuts	175
Millet	162
Rye	115
Tofu	111
Brown rice	88
Soybeans, cooked	88
Dried figs	71
Dried apricots	62
Dates	58
Sunflower seeds	38
Barley	37
Green peas	35
Broccoli	24
Carrot	23
Celery	22

versity of New York Health Sciences Center at Brooklyn, have led the way in establishing the fact that magnesium deprivation is harmful to animal hearts and that magnesium supplementation can make animal hearts healthier. Dr. Altura put a group of rabbits on a high-cholesterol diet. When he deprived them of magnesium, the animals experienced a remarkably accelerated rate of atherosclerosis. They quickly got heart disease. When Dr. Altura then increased the magnesium in the diet of these same animals, their rate of atherosclerosis plummeted. More magnesium was actually good for their arteries and hearts. This result has been replicated many times. Almost invariably, certain high-magnesium diets reduce the development of atherosclerosis in animals, while low magnesium diets accelerate it.

Doctors can't deliberately cause heart disease in humans by depriving them of magnesium, of course. But they've arrived at plenty of other persuasive circumstantial evidence showing what happens to the heart health of healthy people who have low-magnesium diets.

The Atherosclerosis Risk in Communities (ARIC) Study, for instance, which has followed about 15,000 people ages 45 to 64 in four different U.S. communities between 1986 and 1990, reports the danger of low magnesium in our diets. In 1995, the ARIC study found that the less magnesium in people's diets and blood, the higher their insulin, blood sugar, and triglyceride levels and blood pressure and the lower their HDL (high-density lipoprotein, or "good" cholesterol) levels. It also found that women who had lower magnesium levels were also significantly more likely to have thickening of the carotid artery walls of their necks, a sign of plaque buildup that can lead to cerebral stroke. Furthermore, people who had heart disease, hypertension (high blood pressure), and diabetes generally had lower levels of magnesium in their blood than people free of those diseases.

Furthermore, magnesium is known to reduce insulin resistance. There's also a huge amount of medically accepted information around showing that insulin resistance is an independent risk factor for heart disease as well as diabetes. In other words, if magnesium can reduce insulin resistance in healthy people, it should also be able to reduce their incidence of cardiovascular disease.

The research bears this hypothesis out. One study, for example, published in the *New England Journal of Medicine* in 1996, looked at whether there was a connection between high levels of insulin in the blood—a sign of insulin resistance—and ischemic heart disease. It found that even among disease-free people who had low total cholesterol and high HDL cholesterol—in other words, people who had healthy levels of fat in their blood—the higher the insulin levels in their blood, the greater their risk of ischemic heart disease. The connection was even stronger among those who had high total cholesterol and low HDL cholesterol levels.

Here's another piece of admittedly circumstantial evidence. Soft water binds magnesium and makes it unavailable, which means that people living in areas where their drinking water is soft absorb less magnesium than those who drink hard water, even though they may be taking in as much magnesium through their diets. As far back as the 1960s, a number of studies have demonstrated that more people who live in areas with soft water have ischemic heart disease and stroke than people in hard-water areas.

Controlling Blood Pressure

In 1997, the Campbell's Soup Company's Campbell's Center for Nutrition and Wellness decided to test a new, dietetically balanced meal program called Intelligent Quisine. They provided meals that met the dietary guidelines of the American Heart Association and the recommendations of the American Diabetes Association to 563 people at eight universities. The results were impressive. After 10 weeks, 73 percent had lower blood cholesterol levels, 75 percent had lower blood pressure, and 62 percent had lower blood sugar.

The diet included a daily 400- to 450-milligram dose of magnesium in bread products, considerably more than most Americans eat in their food every day. The researchers also found that the more magnesium people had in their bodies—as measured through urinary magnesium excretion—the more their blood pressure fell.

Unfortunately, you can't buy Intelligent Quisine. Campbell's chose to discontinue the program in late 1998 for economic reasons. But you can learn from the impressive results.

How does magnesium lower your blood pressure? One of the country's leading experts on magnesium, Lawrence Resnick, M.D., professor of medicine and director of hypertension at Wayne State University School of Medicine in Detroit, has found that certain people with hypertension tend to have low magnesium inside their cells. They also happen to do very well with magnesium supplementation. "The people with the most circulating angiotensin II," he said in an interview, "got the best results in terms of lowering their blood pressure from taking magnesium."

Angiotensin II, as mentioned earlier, makes your arteries constrict, and magnesium is nature's angiotensin II inhibitor. Dr. Resnick was one of the advisors on Campbell's Intelligent Quisine project and has published numerous independent papers on this subject.

In 1987, the Honolulu Heart Study examined the associations between blood pressure and diet in 615 healthy men of Japanese ancestry living in Hawaii. The researchers looked at 61 different dietary variables, including how much magnesium, calcium, phosphorus, potassium, fiber, vegetable protein, starch, vitamin C, and vitamin D people ingested. Out of all these supplements, magnesium was the most strongly associated with blood pressure. People who supplemented their diets with magnesium fared the best. There was a modest but definite drop in blood pressure compared with those who did not take supplemental magnesium. The association between magnesium in the diet and lower blood pressure held up whether the magnesium came from food or from a supplement.

In a Japanese study that ran in *Hypertension* in 1998, 60 men and women with normal high blood pressure—meaning that they had mild to moderate hypertension—were given either 360 milligrams of magnesium daily or a placebo. After 8 weeks, the blood pressure of the magnesium group dropped by a small but significant amount. Odds are, magnesium was responsible. Concluded the clinical researchers: "Our study supports the usefulness of increasing magnesium intake as a lifestyle modification in the management of hypertension, although its anti-hypertensive effect may be small."

There are, I must add, other studies that do not corroborate these positive results. Dr. Resnick believes that the optimum response occurs in people who already have low intracellular magnesium levels. If the levels are normal, then one cannot expect a response. The information on magnesium's ability to keep your blood pressure normal is not always consistent. But given magnesium's role in your body, the overall direction of research certainly suggests that magnesium supplementation can help keep blood pressure down in some patients.

Magnesium and Congestive Heart Failure

Numerous studies have documented that people who have had heart failure tend to have lower levels of magnesium in their blood and cells than healthy individuals. In part, this is because they frequently take diuretics and drugs such as digoxin, which make them excrete magnesium. But not all people with heart failure take these drugs, and there's still a relatively low level of magnesium in the tissues of this group as a whole.

Here again, magnesium's ability to prevent arrhythmias is largely responsible for its effectiveness in treating people with congestive heart failure. These individuals are particularly susceptible to lethal arrhythmias and sudden death because their condition is, by definition, a weakness in their heart muscle. They also frequently experience nonlethal arrhythmias, wherein their hearts skip beats, beat irregularly, or beat too quickly.

A double-blind study run by a team led by Yaver Bashir, M.D., of the department of cardiological sciences in London's St. George's Hospital Medical School, and published in the *American Journal of Cardiology* in 1993 was one of the first to examine the effect of magnesium on congestive heart failure. These researchers gave 21 people who had congestive heart failure magnesium chloride pills every day for 6 weeks, then a placebo for 6 weeks. The results? Not only did their blood pressure drop significantly but the frequency of their arrhythmias dropped by 23 to 52 percent, depending upon the types of arrhythmias measured.

Others active in the field have corroborated and elaborated on this team's results. One in particular, S. S. Gottlieb, M.D., of the University of Maryland School of Medicine in Baltimore, has demonstrated repeatedly that patients with congestive heart failure tend to have low levels of magnesium in their blood and that giving them magnesium can reduce their arrhythmias.

In one study, Dr. Gottlieb looked at magnesium levels in 199 congestive heart disease patients. He found that the less magnesium they had in their blood, the more severe their arrhythmias, and the lower their blood levels of magnesium, the worse their long-term prognosis.

Could administration of magnesium help such patients? Dr. Gottlieb would say yes. In 1993, his team gave magnesium intravenously to 40 patients with chronic congestive heart failure. Magnesium did not help everyone, but it did effectively treat arrhythmia in patients who were having more than 100 arrhythmic events per hour. And when the researchers measured the level of magnesium in people's blood, they found that whenever the blood magnesium level went up, the frequency of patients' arrhythmias dropped.

The researchers concluded that people with congestive heart failure and low magnesium levels in their blood could benefit from supplemental magnesium, given intravenously.

Even if magnesium can only reduce the incidence of sudden death from heart failure by a small percentage, it's certainly worth considering. In other words, congestive heart failure patients should discuss with their doctors the possibility of supplementing their

(continued on page 160)

Chromium: Elixir Nutraceutical for Diabetes

Magnesium isn't the only supplement that can help reduce the body's resistance to insulin. People with diabetes should consider adding another component to the Cardiac Elixir: chromium, a trace mineral.

Researchers have been looking into the interaction of chromium with insulin for 40 years. Articles describing chromium's potential for helping people with diabetes have been appearing in medical literature since 1977. Chromium seems to help people with diabetes reduce blood sugar and possibly get by on less insulin because, like magnesium, it helps regulate insulin action. And people with diabetes seem to be low in chromium, a situation analogous to magnesium deficiency.

Previously, the proof was limited to very small studies, results that weren't definitive, or clinical research that wasn't rigorous enough to convince medical experts. That's not true any more. Today, chromium's effectiveness in helping reduce insulin sensitivity has achieved medical respectability.

Working with membranes of fat cells or rat liver insulin receptors, one team of researchers demonstrated that chromium acts directly on the cell's insulin receptors. They found that insulin can stimulate enzyme activity by about 60 percent; the addition of chromium resulted in a sevenfold stimulation of the activity.

As for chromium's effect on people, four important clinical studies provide a clear picture.

• The most impressive was published by William Cefalu, M.D., of the department of internal medicine at Bowman Gray School of Medicine of Wake Forest University in Winston–Salem, North Carolina, and others in *Diabetes* and presented to the 1997 annual meeting of the American Diabetes Association. As part of a double-blind placebo–controlled study, he gave 26 overweight people with diabetes either 1,000 micrograms of chromium or a placebo daily for 8 months. He discovered that the sensitivity of their cells to insulin increased by an average of 40 percent. This is known as insulin resistance. Because insulin doesn't function normally, the cells won't let sugar in. And it's an independent risk factor for cardiovascular disease.

• Alexander Ravina, M.D., and his colleagues at the diabetes department of the Lunn Clinic in Haifa, Israel, compared the effect of 200 micrograms of chromium picolinate, the most common form of chromium, with a placebo on 262 people with type 1 (insulin-dependent) and type 2 (non-insulin-dependent) diabetes. The chromium group needed 70 percent less insulin and other blood sugar–regulating medications.

• Richard Anderson, Ph.D., a researcher with the U.S. Department of Agriculture, gave a group of people without diabetes a low-chromium diet, then measured everyone's insulin and glucose levels. People who had normal glucose tolerance showed no effect, but those with poor glucose tolerance got higher sugar and insulin levels in their blood. These effects were partially reversed when Dr. Anderson gave his subjects supplemental chromium.

• Dr. Anderson went on to publish another important study in *Diabetes* in 1997. He led a team of American nutrition scientists and clinicians in three large hospitals in Beijing, China, in a large, double-blind placebo-controlled clinical trial on chromium's effect on people with type 2 diabetes.

Every day for four months, 180 adults with diabetes took either 200 micrograms of chromium picolinate, 1,000 micrograms (1 milligram) of chromium picolinate, or a placebo. Both groups of patients that took chromium supplements enjoyed a significant drop in both blood sugar and blood insulin levels. Dr. Anderson also reported that the group receiving the larger dose of chromium had a drop in their blood cholesterol levels as well.

The researchers pointed out that chromium had this effect because of its ability to help insulin work. By decreasing insulin sensitivity, it reduced the resistance of cells to insulin and helped insulin move glucose into the cells. In other words, people with diabetes who take chromium may require much lower levels of insulin and not only have better glucose metabolism but also lower risk factors associated with cardiovascular disease. In a follow-up study published in 1998, the researchers confirmed these results.

(continued)

Chromium: Elixir Nutraceutical for Diabetes—Continued

Why supplement with chromium?

Once you know the available sources, you'll realize that you'll probably have to supplement. Your best source of chromium is brewer's yeast, hardly a gourmet delight. Other good sources of chromium are liver, egg yolks, broccoli, whole-grain cereals, bran, wheat germ, and oysters. Notice that none of these are refined foods like flour and sugar—the mainstay of many an American diet. Foods high in sugars are not only low in chromium but they can actually deplete your body's chromium stores. According to the USDA, chromium is more likely to be in short supply in the average American diet than any other vitamin or mineral.

How much should you take?

Dr. Anderson discovered that the amount of chromium that his subjects required depended on their level of glucose intolerance. People with diabetes who were mildly glucose intolerant did well on 200 micrograms daily, while those who had high levels of glucose intolerance needed up to 1,000 micrograms daily.

An important note on supplementation for people with diabetes: Work with your doctor. Diabetes is a serious disease that requires day-to-day attention. Be sure to tell your doctor if you are considering taking chromium.

medications with magnesium. An estimated four million patients in the United States have congestive heart failure. This number is rapidly increasing because of our aging population. For this reason alone, more attention should be paid to magnesium.

The Diabetes Connection

Diabetes has become a serious and endemic health problem in this country. There are approximately nine million people with diabetes in the United States and millions more that are undiagnosed. According to a report released in 1999 by the Diabetes Research Working Group, a group appointed by Congress to develop plans for diabetes research, the mortality rate from this disease has increased 30 percent since 1980. It now kills one American every 3 minutes.

What do people with diabetes die of?

Much of the time, ischemic heart disease is responsible. Insulin resistance, as you've already learned, is an independent risk factor for heart disease. People with diabetes are twice as likely to have heart attacks due to coronary artery disease as the rest of the population and two to five times more likely to have strokes, congestive heart failure, major arterial disease, or hypertension. Some 60 to 70 percent of people with type 2 (adult-onset, or non-insulin-dependent) diabetes will die of any one of these manifestations of heart disease.

One reason that doctors will tell you why people with diabetes are vulnerable to cardiovascular problems is because their disease has an interrelated complex of manifestations—called Syndrome X—that make it much harder for their bodies to transport enough oxygen to their tissues. The manifestations of Syndrome X include:

- *Plaque formation in the big vessels, such as the aorta, carotid artery, and large arteries in the arms and legs*

- *Circulatory problems due to blockages in the smaller arteries and their branches; these can lead to complications such as gangrene*

- *Insulin resistance*

- *Higher blood triglyceride levels than the general population*

- *Low levels of LDL (the good cholesterol) in the blood*

- *High blood sugar*

- *Hypertension (high blood pressure)*

- *Increased blood clotting*

■ *Increased sensitivity to angiotensin II, the hormone your kidneys produce that constricts blood vessels*

■ *Obesity, mostly around the abdominal area*

If you reread the list of symptoms for Syndrome X, you may experience a feeling of déjà vu. Many of them are the exact manifestations of magnesium deficiency that were discussed in the first half of this chapter.

Indeed, clinical studies have demonstrated that most people with diabetes, both insulin-dependent and non-insulin-dependent, also have a deficiency of magnesium inside their cells. In 1979, a researcher by the name of Dr. H. M. Mather found that patients who suffered from diabetes had significantly lower levels of magnesium inside their cells than people who did not suffer from diabetes. And these results have been replicated many times since then here in the United States and internationally. Let's discuss just two of them.

■ *Robert Rude, M.D., of the University of Southern California in Los Angeles, who served as the magnesium expert for the National Academy of Sciences panel in 1997, published a study that measured the free levels of magnesium in the white blood cells of people without diabetes and people with the disease. He discovered that if you incubate the cells of healthy people with insulin, the insulin can attach itself to the cells, and the amount of glucose as well as magnesium in those cells goes up. If you incubate the cells of people with diabetes—cells that are insulin-resistant— the amount of glucose and magnesium inside the cell is measurably lower.*

■ *Another intriguing study was conducted by an Italian clinical researcher, Guisseppe Paolisso, M.D., who is very active in this field. He compared the amount of intracellular magnesium in the cells of Pima tribespeople native to Arizona, who are known to be insulin-resistant, with the amount in the cells of healthy Caucasians. The cells from the Pima tribespeople took in less glucose and also had lower levels of magnesium.*

The Benefits for Diabetes

No one knows which came first—the diabetes or the magnesium deficiency.

But an exciting body of research strongly suggests that supplementation with magnesium can almost certainly help prevent or maybe even treat insulin resistance and other cardiovascular problems in people with diabetes.

As I mentioned earlier in this chapter, I've been convinced of the importance of magnesium for people with diabetes for some time. I helped coordinate a consensus group of medical experts on the role of magnesium supplementation in the treatment of diabetes with the American Diabetes Association way back in 1992. The experts concluded that the weight of experimental data suggests that magnesium deficiency may well play a role in insulin resistance, carbohydrate intolerance, and high blood pressure.

In other words, when there is magnesium deficiency in a patient with diabetes, it should be corrected. There are even more data now, and the story is becoming even more compelling.

What's the connection between magnesium and diabetes? Why are people with diabetes prone to magnesium deficiency? Though there are many theories, no one knows. What is important to note is that many people with diabetes eat various types of food but still

A Chromium Profile

What it is:
A trace mineral found in most of your cells

What it does:
It can help reduce insulin resistance, which is an important cardiovascular risk factor; it may lower blood sugar

Mechanism of protection:
By reducing insulin resistance, it may have a beneficial effect on myocardial ischemia and myocardial infarctions or heart attacks.

Where you can buy it:
Pharmacies, health food stores, and supermarkets

What to look for on the label:
Chromium picolinate

Who it's for:
People with diabetes

How much to take:
500 to 1,000 micrograms, or ½ to 1 milligram

are magnesium-deficient. This strengthens the argument for supplementation as the best way to replete the body's stores. Magnesium can help people with diabetes in a number of ways.

Magnesium can reduce insulin resistance. As I stated earlier, clinical researchers have uncovered a correlation between insulin resistance and magnesium deficiency. The cells of practically all people with diabetes are insulin-resistant. And insulin resistance is closely connected with many of the cardiovascular problems endemic to people with diabetes. People with insulin resistance are more prone to many of the manifestations of Syndrome X such as high blood pressure, impaired blood clotting, accumulation of excess fat in blood, and atherosclerosis.

More than one study has concluded that people with insulin resistance also have low levels of magnesium in their tissues and that magnesium supplementation can reduce insulin resistance. When Dr. Nadler and his colleagues put 16 healthy people on magnesium-deficient diets for a mere 3 weeks, for instance, their cells not only became deficient in magnesium but the insulin of every single individual became less capable of transporting sugar from the blood into the cells. He discussed these results to the attendees at my November 1997 Foundation for Innovation in Medicine (FIM) conference and made these provocative remarks: "You can induce insulin resistance even in people who do not have diabetes. Just deprive them of magnesium."

Nine small studies have tested the effect of 360 milligrams to 390 milligrams of magnesium per day over 1 to 5 months. Although six of these studies found that the magnesium had no effect on lowering people's blood sugar, three did find that the magnesium improved their insulin sensitivity. I'm not surprised by these results. Magnesium is not likely to change blood sugar very much, but it may improve insulin sensitivity, which may improve long-term prospects of avoiding a heart attack or stroke in people with diabetes.

Magnesium can reduce blood clotting. As part of Syndrome X, people with diabetes are prone to excessive blood clotting, a risk factor for dangerous plaque buildup and artery blockages. Indeed, Dr. Nadler has discovered that people with type 2 diabetes, in addition to being magnesium-deficient, also have double the amount of the blood-clotting factor thromboxane compared to people without diabetes. Magnesium supplementation, Dr. Nadler says, may help reduce vascular disease in patients with diabetes by reducing their thromboxane levels

Magnesium may help some people who are diabetic manage high blood pressure. Magnesium's potential to help control blood pressure is especially important for people with diabetes. Dr. Resnick and his colleagues measured magnesium levels in people with non-insulin-dependent diabetes and in people without diabetes. He found that those people with diabetes who had significantly lower magnesium levels also had higher blood pressure than people without the disease. He also found that all his subjects with high blood pressure, whether diabetic or nondiabetic, had lower magnesium levels than people with normal blood pressure. A follow-up study confirmed these results.

Exactly how does magnesium keep blood pressure down for people with diabetes who have low levels of intracellular magnesium? It probably reduces the sensitivity of these people to angiotensin II—the hormone produced by the kidneys that makes blood vessels clamp down. Here again, there's good clinical evidence that magnesium can help. Dr. Resnick has discovered that people with low levels of angiotensin II are high in magnesium, and those with excessive amounts of angiotensin II are low in magnesium. "I have treated people who were hypertensive and on one or two medications with magnesium," says Dr. Resnick. "Their blood pressure is now normal."

If you have diabetes, you probably don't know if your cells are deficient in magnesium, though it's highly likely. Routine laboratory tests do not include blood and intracellular magnesium levels. Until such time, it is wise for people with diabetes, with certain exceptions such as those with kidney disease, to take daily supplementation of this mineral.

Just a brief note of caution here: Don't ever replace any blood pressure medications with magnesium or any nutraceutical without discussing this possibility with your physician.

An Early Warning System for Diabetes

If you don't have diabetes, don't get complacent. There's good evidence that low levels of magnesium in your body could be an early warning sign that you may one day contract diabetes, along with its concomitant cardiovascular risks.

Earlier in this chapter, when I mentioned the ARIC (Atherosclerosis Risk in Communities) study, you learned that low magnesium levels can be correlated to a whole host of cardiovascular disease risk factors in healthy people. The clinical researchers didn't stop there. In 1997, the ARIC researchers updated their findings with a new paper. People who had the lowest levels of magnesium in their blood at the beginning of the study were twice as likely to be diagnosed later with diabetes as those with the highest levels of magnesium, according to Frederick Brancati, M.D., an epidemiologist at the Johns Hopkins University School of Medicine in Baltimore. This twofold risk of developing diabetes was independent of every other risk factor that can cause diabetes.

The Nurses' Health Study has been following the diets and health of 85,000 nurses since 1976, and the Prospective Health Professionals study, also known has the Health Professionals Follow-Up Study, has likewise been done for tens of thousands of male health professionals since 1986. Both studies revealed a significant connection between magnesium intake and the risk of developing diabetes in healthy people. The Nurses' Health Study found that women who consumed about 220 milligrams of magnesium daily were about one-third more likely to develop diabetes over the next 6 years than those who consumed about 340 milligrams daily. The more magnesium these women took in, the lower their risk of getting diabetes. The Prospective Health Professionals Study showed similar results.

Clearly, it could be in your interest to keep your magnesium levels up, particularly if you have a family history of diabetes.

Why It's Important to Supplement

You may be thinking that you'd better head off to your doctor and see whether you're magnesium-deficient. Certainly, the consensus group held by the American Diabetes Association has recommended that doctors measure the magnesium levels of high-risk patients, such as alcoholics, pregnant women, those taking drugs that could lead to magnesium deficiency, or those who had had heart failure or a recent heart attack. Their position was and is that if these tests uncover a magnesium deficiency, doctors should advise their patients to correct it through diet or supplements.

The trouble is that most hospitals do not routinely measure your magnesium levels. Even among those who do, the standard tests for magnesium may not reveal the whole truth. Most tests measure the amount of magnesium that's in your blood serum (the fluid, excluding the blood cells). But this serum only contains about 1 percent of the magnesium in your body. The other 99 percent of your body's magnesium is inside your cells. You can have so-called normal amounts of magnesium in your blood serum and still be magnesium-deficient inside your cells, which is where it really matters. Unless your doctor specifically orders tests on your intracellular level of magnesium, you'll never know the truth.

People with diabetes are particularly vulnerable to this type of misdiagnosis. In one study, for instance, Dr. Resnick compared the magnesium levels in about 30 people without diabetes and that of people with type 2 diabetes. He found little differences in total serum magnesium between the two groups. It was only when he used rather sophisticated techniques to compare the level of magnesium inside their cells that he could see a difference. "Most diabetics have intracellular magnesium deficiency," he said in an interview. "But if you look for it in their blood, you'll find that 70 to 80 percent have normal serum levels."

Dr. Nadler agrees. In his studies conducted at the University of Southern California in Los Angeles, the total magnesium wasn't substantially different between people with and without diabetes. But about 80 to 90 percent of the patients had low intracellular free magnesium. A dose of oral magnesium for 6 weeks reversed this.

"Along with many other studies, we confirmed that type 2 diabetics tend to have low intracellular free magnesium," Dr. Nadler says. "We also demonstrated that you can replete or correct this by supplementation."

Diet Is Not Enough

Theoretically, you can get magnesium from eating dairy products, whole-grain products, unprocessed vegetables, legumes, nuts, and soy products. Drinking water can also contribute somewhat to your total magnesium intake if you live in an area where the water is hard.

In practice, though, most people can't get enough magnesium from their food. How many people do you know that live primarily on unprocessed, whole-grain products? In the early 1900s, when people did eat more natural food products, they ingested 475 to 500 milligrams of magnesium in their food daily. Today, it's an average of 143 to 266 milligrams per day—well below what you need for a cardiac health strategy.

Take a look at "Sources of Magnesium in Your Diet," on page 152. Are you getting enough magnesium from your diet? I doubt it. As for drinking water, there are only 3 to 20 milligrams of magnesium in each liter. You would have to literally drink a bathtub full of water every day to raise your magnesium levels.

To compound the difficulty of getting enough magnesium in your diet, magnesium isn't usually listed on food-packaging labels, so you can't monitor your magnesium intake on your own, even if you wanted to.

How Much Should You Take?

Dr. Rude—the doctor who served as the magnesium expert for the National Academy of Sciences (NAS) panel in 1997—strongly recommends that we increase our official minimum requirements for magnesium intake. Largely because of his input, the NAS today suggests that women over age 30 consume 320 milligrams of magnesium daily, while men should consume at least 420 milligrams daily.

To be on the conservative side, I recommend that you take 400 to 450 milligrams of magnesium daily. That will ensure that you're getting enough.

You can find magnesium in a variety of forms, including magnesium oxide, magnesium chloride, magnesium gluconate, magnesium animo acids chelate (chelated magnesium), and magnesium carbonate. Ask your pharmacist or physician which forms are absorbed best.

CHAPTER ELEVEN

Alcohol for Heart Health

Each night before dinner, my wife and I usually enjoy a buen trago, or cocktail, together, and talk about the events of the day. It's our way of relaxing after the day's work.

There is little doubt that drinking in moderation is good for your cardiovascular health. Alcohol is the most thoroughly studied nutraceutical in the Cardiac Elixir. Since the 1970s, more than 70 clinical studies have consistently found that people who have one or two drinks a day have, on average, a 30 to 40 percent lower risk of dying of heart disease than nondrinkers. It doesn't seems to matter whether you drink wine, beer, or spirits such as gin, vodka, or bourbon. They all seem to confer protection against heart disease.

The dangers of too much alcohol are well-known. As a physician, I feel compelled to underline the risks. They are quite real. Just a few of its many downsides are listed in "Cautionary Words on the Cardiovascular Dangers of Alcohol" on page 172. Exces-

170

sive drinking can damage your heart and your liver and put you at higher risk for some cancers, not to mention destroy your marriage and your job.

The Persian philosopher Zoroaster perceived the world as a battleground between good and evil. Alcohol embodies that tension. Too much can be both a physical and mental health hazard, but just enough can make life more pleasurable and significantly reduce coronary artery disease. Moderation is the key word. This is one nutraceutical where getting the right dose is very important.

A Powerful, Fast-Acting Agent

Alcohol is a chemical compound created by the fermentation of grapes, apples, grains, and other plants. People have been drinking it in various forms for ages, not to protect their hearts but to numb their pain and boost spirits. Sigmund Freud was right when he said that life is tough and we all need our palliatives. There is even evidence that animals have a taste for alcohol. Some naturalists have theorized that elephants like to eat fermented bananas for the intoxication effect.

Unlike food, alcohol doesn't have to pass through your stomach and into your intestines for your body to absorb it. Rather, it diffuses through the walls of your stomach directly into your bloodstream. Once there, it goes quickly to your brain and often induces a pleasant feeling of well-being, confidence, and cheer.

But even as alcohol is making you feel "high," it's actually functioning as a depressant, slowing down your central nervous system. That's why your muscles relax, your reflexes slow, and you end up feeling sleepy. In fact, before the advent of modern anesthetics, people used alcohol to deaden pain. But aside from these depressing effects on your brain, alcohol in the right dose has many positive effects on your circulatory system.

Alcohol increases your high-density lipoproteins. Remember them? Your high-density lipoproteins (HDLs) are the "good guys" that

Cautionary Words on the Cardiovascular Dangers of Alcohol

Since time began, preachers and doctors have been warning about the risks of demon rum. There's plenty of good reason to rant and rave. Even though alcohol can reduce the occurrence of heart disease in the general population, it can also cause harm, including harm to the cardiovascular system.

Simply put, only in moderation can alcohol enhance your health and your life.

Here's just a small sampling of some of the problems that too much of a good thing can lead to.

• Too much of that pleasant, relaxed, and comfortable feeling has a down side. People who drink to excess can be prone to obesity and an excessively sedentary lifestyle—both of which put you at increased risk of heart disease and cancel out alcohol's heart benefits.

• Alcohol has a myocardial depressant effect. This is a sophisticated way of saying that it can weaken the pumping action of your heart's left ventricle, thus depriving your body of the oxygen and other nutrients carried by your blood.

•Too much alcohol will literally make it hard for your body to fight off infection because it inhibits your immune system. It puts you at higher risk for many different diseases.

• Alcohol's ability to inhibit your platelets is dangerous for binge drinkers, who could fall down in a drunken stupor and suffer uncontrolled internal bleeding or a hemorrhagic stroke (a stroke in the brain caused by cerebral bleeding).

carry cholesterol away from the inner lining of your arteries and back into your liver for elimination or reprocessing.

As far back as 1983, researchers have known that even relatively small amounts of alcohol, such as 40 grams daily, increased people's

• Although alcohol in moderate amounts lowers your blood pressure, it can cause high blood pressure in higher amounts. And high blood pressure is a major risk factor for stroke.

• Alcohol depletes your body's supply of magnesium. The effect may play a role in raising the blood pressure of binge drinkers. If you're a moderate drinker who takes magnesium as part of your cardiovascular elixir, this particular side effect may not hit you too hard.

• Alcohol abuse wreaks havoc on people's digestive systems as well as other vital organs. Your liver, which is responsible for detoxifying alcohol in your body, can be severely damaged. Also, alcohol abuse accounts for most of the cases of pancreatitis in this country.

• If you drink too much, you may not be consuming enough of the foods—or nutraceuticals—that you need. Too much alcohol interferes with the activity of most vitamins and some nutrients, including iron, thiamin, folate, vitamin A, and zinc.

• Alcoholism or long-term binge drinking—drinking to the point of extreme intoxication repeatedly—can cause heart failure (your heart becomes too weak to pump) or arrhythmias. Binge drinking can also give you liver failure, even dementia. You could suffer neuromuscular impairment so severe that you'd be prone to dangerous falls.

• If you already have heart disease—particularly, myocardial ischemia (shortage of oxygen to the heart muscle) or congestive heart failure—you may well be prone to arrhythmias even if you drink minimal amounts of alcohol.

• Alcohol can also cause congestive cardiomyopathy, an ailment that frequently strikes men ranging from ages 30 to 55 if they have consumed 30 to 50 percent of their total calories as alcohol for 10 or more years.

HDL levels by up to 17 percent within 6 weeks. And as you've already learned, a relatively high ratio of HDL compared with low-density lipoprotein (LDL, or "bad" cholesterol) in your bloodstream is associated with fewer cholesterol deposits in your arteries and hence, protection against atherosclerosis. It is estimated that a 17 percent increase of HDLs could account for up to a 40 percent reduction in your risk of developing heart disease.

Exactly how alcohol increases your HDL level is still under investigation. Some researchers think that alcohol may, in effect, signal your liver and intestines to make more of the proteins that your body needs to make its HDLs. But there may be other physiological forces in play. More research will eventually uncover the mechanism.

In any case, no one disputes this effect because it has been demonstrated in study after study. In 1993, for instance, J. Michael Gaziano, M.D., and others of the Brigham and Women's Hospital in Boston, published a study in the *New England Journal of Medicine* looking at the connection between alcohol consumption, blood lipoprotein levels, and heart attack risk in 340 men and women who had already had heart attacks. It found that the more people drank, the higher their levels of HDL cholesterol and the less at risk they were of another heart attack.

Alcohol slows down platelet aggregation and fibrinogen formation. This means that drinking can decrease the tendency of your blood to clot. It likely does this by increasing the level of a major clot-dissolving enzyme called tissue plasminogen activator (t-PA). And blood clots are an important component of plaque. A clot can also block off an entire artery, which can trigger a heart attack if it's in the coronary artery or a stroke if it's in the carotid artery.

Alcohol may lower insulin resistance. Resistance to insulin is a major risk factor for cardiovascular disease and heart attacks, both for people with diabetes and those without. Research suggests that moderate amounts of alcohol seem to help insulin coax glucose into your cells, keeping it from pooling in your bloodstream and damaging your blood vessels.

It's important to note that all these beneficial effects can prevent atherosclerosis. Alcohol is good for your heart only because it helps keep your arteries free of plaque. Sometimes, though, it's not good for your actual heart muscle. (See "Cautionary Words on the Cardiovascular Dangers of Alcohol" on page 172.)

An Alcohol Profile

What it is:

Any alcoholic beverage, including wine, beer, and spirits

What it does:

Increases your "good" high-density lipoprotein (HDL) cholesterol levels and slows down blood clotting

Mechanism of protection:

Prevents plaque and clot formation in your arteries

Where you can buy it:

Liquor stores, grocery and convenience stores in some states, beverage distributors, and bars

What to look for on the label:

Not applicable, as labels typically do not list product composition; all types of alcohol provide protection

Who it's for:

It is illegal for anyone under a state's legal age requirement to drink (that age is 21 in most states); however, alcohol in moderate quantities provides protective health benefits to adults of legal age; recommended for healthy people, people who have coronary artery disease, people with myocardial ischemia or angina, people at risk of ischemic stroke, and people who have had a heart attack

Who it's *not* for:

Anyone with a genetic susceptibility to alcoholism or binge drinking, or anyone who has a moral or religious objection or cardiomyopathy or a blood-clotting disorder; if you're on any medications, double-check with your doctor; alcohol is not recommended for pregnant women

How much to drink:

For its protective effect on your heart, approximately one to two drinks daily for men, one drink daily for women; a drink is a 12-ounce bottle of beer or a wine cooler, a 4- to 5-ounce glass of wine, or 1¼ to 1½ ounces of 80-proof distilled spirits.

The Evidence for Heart Protection

Twice every year, my Foundation for Innovation in Medicine (FIM) sponsors a conference on nutraceuticals to discuss the latest developments in the field. During our November 1997 conference on cardiovascular nutraceuticals, one of the featured speakers was George Schreiner, M.D., Ph.D., an internationally respected researcher who is vice president of Cardiorenal Research for Scios in Sunnyvale, California. His research group decided to look at the overall results of as many studies as possible examining the possible connections between alcohol and heart disease risk. They analyzed 30 different studies published between 1968 and 1993. Many thousands of men and women belonging to a wide variety of racial and ethnic groups from around the world participated in these studies.

Dr. Schreiner reported that 24 out of these 30 studies demonstrated that people who drank alcohol were statistically less likely to get coronary artery disease. Exactly what benefit did the subjects enjoy? Their protection ranged from 29 percent less likely to get cardiovascular disease all the way up to 70 percent less likely. The numbers varied, depending upon the amount of alcohol that people drank and the categories of cardiovascular disease risk specific to each research team.

The vast majority of these studies pointed in exactly the same direction. Alcohol produced a marked reduction in cardiovascular disease rates, whether the researchers defined disease as ischemia, heart attacks, the need for angioplasty, the need for bypass surgery, the incidence of fatal arrhythmias, or the incidence of strokes. This consistent finding in studies both large-scale and small continues to this day.

As you've already learned, Harvard University is involved in a number of very large studies looking at the effects of many components of our diets. They include the Health Professionals Follow-Up Study, which has been tracking the dietary habits and health of more than 50,000 male health professionals since 1986; the Physicians' Health Study, which has been following more than 20,000 physicians since 1984; and the Nurses' Health Study, which has been looking at the health of more than 80,000 women since 1980. All of these groups have independently discovered clear connections between alcohol and heart health.

In 1988, Meir Stampfer, M.D., Dr.P.H., professor of epidemi-ology and nutrition at the Harvard School of Public Health, and his group published their first study of alcohol consumption and risk of coronary disease in women. The study found a definite cor-relation between moderate alcohol consumption and reduced risk of heart disease in women. Improbable as it may seem, even women who have as little as one drink a week reportedly experience a 50 percent reduction in risk. Women do seem to require less alcohol than men for heart protection, but I'd like to deal with that issue in more detail later on in this chapter.

In 1991, Eric Rimm, Sc.D., assistant professor of nutrition and epidemiology at the Harvard School of Public Health, and his group published an important study of alcohol consumption and risk of coronary disease in men. Even after adjustment for coronary risk factors such as high-cholesterol, low-fiber diets, the researchers found that men who drank up to three to four drinks daily enjoyed up to 30 percent less risk of heart disease.

Next up was the Physicians' Health Study, led by a team of re-searchers from Boston's Brigham and Women's Hospital and Har-vard Medical School, under a group led by Carlos A. Camargo Jr., M.D. They published their findings in the American Heart Associ-ation's *Archives of Internal Medicine* in 1997. The results confirmed the beneficial effects of alcohol.

Dr. Camargo's group discovered that men who drank moder-ately (one to six drinks weekly) were healthier overall than those it defined as heavy drinkers (two or more drinks daily) or light drinkers (less than one drink weekly). Healthy men who con-sumed one drink daily were 31 percent less likely to get angina or a heart attack. In a separate analysis, they found that moderate al-cohol consumption also decreased the risk of peripheral arterial disease, which is atherosclerosis of the arteries of the legs, by around 25 percent.

Notice that the beneficial amount to drink varies from person to person and sometimes even from study to study. Dr. Rimm's study found that people who have three to four drinks daily are less at risk of heart disease, while Dr. Camargo's study suggests that healthy men who take two or more drinks daily are less healthy overall than those who consume one drink daily. The bottom line is that the beneficial effect of alcohol in reducing heart disease is consistent. But remember, the more you drink, the more you're at risk of the other negative effects of alcohol.

Fighting Stroke: The Brain Benefits

Theoretically, if alcohol can help prevent plaque formation in your coronary arteries, reducing your risk of heart disease, it should also help prevent plaque formation in the carotid arteries of your neck and reduce your risk of stroke. The clinical evidence supports the theory.

The prestigious *Journal of the American Medical Association* published an important study in early 1999 demonstrating the beneficial possibilities of moderate alcohol consumption on an ischemic stroke (the type of stroke caused by blockage of the brain arteries). It was called the Northern Manhattan Stroke Study, and in it, Ralph L. Sacco, M.D., of the department of neurology at the Serglevky Center at Columbia University College of Physicians and Surgeons in New York City, and his team compared the alcohol intake of 667 New York City residents who had had strokes between 1993 and 1997 with 1,139 other residents who had not had strokes. The subjects were adults over the age of 40, and they were a true multicultural mix—Whites, Blacks, and Hispanics.

During the 4-year period of the study, Dr. Sacco's team found that people who consumed up to two drinks daily were at 45 percent lower risk of having a clot-type stroke than nondrinkers. This protection was found in subjects of varying ages and in every racial group that participated in the study after taking into account differences in other factors that affect stroke risk, such as high blood pressure, cardiac disease, diabetes, smoking, and obesity. It didn't matter whether they drank beer, wine, or other alcohol.

Why Are Women Getting More Heart Disease?

In general, women are at lower risk of heart disease than men, at least until they reach menopause. Why? Probably because their estrogen protects them. After menopause, those who continue taking estrogen in the form of hormone replacement therapy continue to enjoy its beneficial effect on their hearts.

The Framingham Heart Study, a long-term study of virtually the entire population of this small city in Massachusetts, reported that women were considerably less likely than men to get heart disease. But it was also true that women had less stress in their lives than men at the time this study was conducted, and their lower stress levels contributed to their lower incidence of heart disease in that study. Today, increasing numbers of women have exactly the same stress levels as men in their lives, both at home and at work. Their heart disease rates reflect this change; they're rapidly starting to catch up.

One important caveat: The study showed that excessive alcohol had exactly the opposite effect. Once people started downing seven drinks or more daily, their risk of stroke actually went up. In fact, it tripled.

The authors pointed out that there is no evidence that people who don't drink will benefit from taking up alcohol for its potential health benefits. However, their own study supports the view that alcohol consumption among moderate drinkers may reduce the risk of ischemic stroke.

Prevent the Second Heart Attack

In his keynote speech at the 70th Annual Scientific Sessions of the American Heart Association in 1997, Dr. Gaziano discussed a study of the relationship between light to moderate alcohol intake and mortality among men who had reported a previous heart attack or stroke. The study, led by Dr. Jorg Muntwyler, of the department of medicine at Brigham and Women's Hospital and Harvard Medical School, looked at 6,000 male physicians who had originally responded to the Physicians' Health Study in 1981. Dr. Gaziano was a member of Dr. Muntwyler's team.

In this high-risk population, moderate alcohol intake lowered the risk of dying of a second heart attack, cardiovascular disease, or any other cause related or unrelated to heart disease. The more their alcohol intake increased, the higher their odds of staying healthy. The men who took one or more drinks every day reduced their odds by about 30 percent—a figure that sounds remarkably similar to the results of many of the other studies on the alcohol-cardiac link.

The investigators concluded that light to moderate alcohol intake in this large group of people who had had prior heart attacks could protect them from another event and reduce the odds of death.

Even better, Dr. Camargo and his team—the group that discovered how beneficial alcohol can be in preventing angina or a heart attack—also found that the risk of dying from all causes, including cardiovascular diseases, cancer, and other ailments, was 28 percent lower in men who drank two to four drinks weekly and 21 percent lower in men who drank five to six drinks weekly. The alcohol group was 34 to 53 percent less likely to die of cardiovascular disease.

At higher levels of consumption, alcohol turned toxic. The risk of dying was 51 percent higher in heavy drinkers—not from heart disease, but from cancer. The researchers concluded that two to six drinks per week offered the greatest potential benefits.

Women and Alcohol: Why Gender Matters

Though alcohol offers women effective cardiovascular protection, women process alcohol somewhat differently than men and seem to require less of it for cardiac protection.

When you drink alcohol, your stomach secretes an enzyme called dehydrogenase, which breaks down as much as 20 percent of the alcohol and prevents it from entering your bloodstream. Since women produce less of this enzyme than men, they absorb a higher percentage of the alcohol that they drink. If a man and a woman who are the same size have identical glasses of wine, the woman gets a higher effective dose of alcohol. Add in the man-woman size disparity, and the same drink translates into a much higher blood ethanol level for a 130-pound woman than it does for a 180-pound man.

Finally, women's higher body fat content plays a role in alcohol metabolism. The alcohol molecule is absorbed primarily by the body's water spaces, not its fat spaces. Because most women have significantly more body fat content and less water content in their bodies than men, they have less place to store the alcohol, so more of it is absorbed by their bloodstream.

All of these gender differences add up to the fact that women need lower doses of alcohol to get both alcohol's cardiovascular benefits and its related health risks.

On top of this, women seem to process alcohol differently than men. A study done by William Kannel, M.D., of Boston University School of Medicine, and his colleagues demonstrates some of the differences between the genders. They analyzed the Framingham Heart Study, a 24-year-long look at the same population in Framingham, Massachusetts, specifically to assess the incidence of heart disease among men and women, both smokers and nonsmokers. Here's some of what they found.

Among Men

■ *Abstainers were more at risk for heart disease than those who drank moderate amounts of alcohol.*

■ *Drinking even protected the hearts of smokers. Most likely to die of heart disease were the smokers who didn't drink. When the smokers drank, even as little as an ounce of alcohol a week, their risk dropped to that of nonsmoking abstainers.*

■ *Overall, the more the men drank, the less likely they were to die of heart disease. This held true all the way up to 19 drinks a week.*

■ *The men enjoyed a beneficial effect starting at 1 ounce weekly. Nonsmokers were able to cut their risk in half by increasing their consumption from two to three drinks weekly up to four to seven drinks a week.*

Among Women

■ *Women were far less likely to die of heart disease in the first place, whether they drank or not and whether they smoked or not. Only one woman died of heart disease for every three men who did.*

■ *Alcohol protected women just as effectively as it protected men, but it took a smaller dose to do it. Nonsmoking women could significantly lower their risk of dying of heart disease with just 2 to 3 ounces per week (which translates into about half a drink a day). Their smoking sisters could slash their risk of heart disease almost in half by taking a mere ounce of alcohol per week.*

■ *For women, alcohol offered especially strong protection against angina pectoris, chest pain that occurs due to myocardial ischemia, or lack of oxygen to the heart.*

Is Alcohol Riskier for Women?

One particular risk for women that may be associated with alcohol consumption is breast cancer.

In 1998, the *Journal of the American Medical Association* published a study that suggested that regular alcohol consumption may increase the risk of breast cancer. The researcher analyzed six previous studies and found that women who drank, on average, about two to five drinks daily had a 41 percent higher risk of breast cancer than nondrinkers.

Though the level of alcohol in this study is high, these findings present some cause for concern. Other studies have found an increased breast cancer risk at lower alcohol levels. One study that followed 300,000 women for up to 11 years revealed a rise in breast cancer risk when women drank only a glass of wine or a bottle a beer a day.

I don't mean to minimize the findings of all these studies, but it's important to understand the results in context. A woman has about a 12.5 percent chance of developing breast cancer over her lifetime. This study found that one drink increased that risk to 13.4 percent. In contrast, another research team, at Boston University, analyzed the breast cancer risk and drinking habits of two generations of 5,000 women from the Framingham Heart Study and their offspring. Their results, published in early 1999, concluded that women who consume small amounts of alcohol are not at increased risk of developing breast cancer.

Despite these results, I believe that the overall evidence is strong that women, too, can benefit from taking a drink a day. But the fact is that alcohol is a case where the medical truth is still emerging. So it's especially important that you work closely with your doctor in making a judgment about whether to use this nutraceutical.

If you have risk factors for breast cancer, including a powerful family history, you may want to forgo alcohol. If, on the other hand, you don't have high risk factors for breast cancer, but do have some for heart disease, you're probably better off having the drink a day and getting the nutraceutical cardiovascular protection of alcohol.

Of course, if you have risk factors for both diseases or for neither, this is a tougher call. Though all women are at greater risk for heart disease than they are for breast cancer, breast cancer often strikes at an earlier age. I believe that for most women, the cardiac health benefits of minimal alcohol consumption outweigh the possible risk.

How can you decide whether the risks of drinking alcohol in moderation outweigh the heart benefits? Some studies have shown that even moderate drinking may increase your risk of dying of cancer or other diseases. Is it worth the risk? A team of U.S. researchers led by Michael Thun, M.D., of the American Cancer Society, decided to find out. They conducted an investigation of 490,000 men and women ages 35 to 69 who were participants in a huge national study done under the sponsorship of the American Cancer Society. They tracked the health and alcohol consumption of these individuals for 9 years, and they came up with a number of important conclusions.

■ *Those who drank at least one drink daily were 21 percent less likely to die of any cause than nondrinkers.*

■ *The rates of death were lowest among people who took one drink daily. After one drink daily, the rate of death from all causes reported, which included cardiac mortality as well as other ailments, such as cancer, increased with alcohol consumption.*

■ *Daily drinkers were 30 to 40 percent less likely to die of any form of heart disease. The largest reduction occurred in death from coronary heart disease among drinkers who had been suffering from heart disease, stroke, or some other risk factor at the outset of the study.*

■ *Drinking is no panacea for smokers, who were 40 percent more likely than nonsmokers to die from all causes. This study found that alcohol's protection was not enough to offset the health risks of cigarette smoking, taking all possible causes of death or illness into consideration. Smoking is certainly bad for your overall health, but several other major studies clearly indicate that alcohol can help offset the risks of smoking to your heart health specifically.*

Not surprisingly, the researchers also found that heavy drinking was associated with many health problems, including accidents and suicides. On the specific question of cancer, they got two troubling results: (1) Even moderate drinkers were more likely than nondrinkers to die from cirrhosis of the liver or from cancers of the mouth, throat, esophagus, pharynx, larynx, or liver; and (2) women who ingested at least a drink every day faced a 30 percent higher risk of death from breast cancer.

All these risks don't necessarily offset alcohol's potential benefit

The Alcohol You Need

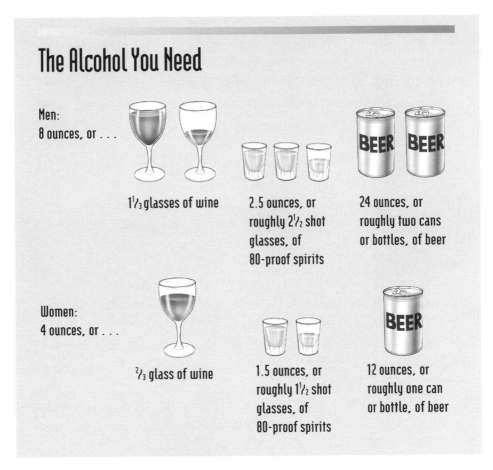

Men:
8 ounces, or . . .

1⅓ glasses of wine

2.5 ounces, or roughly 2½ shot glasses, of 80-proof spirits

24 ounces, or roughly two cans or bottles, of beer

Women:
4 ounces, or . . .

⅔ glass of wine

1.5 ounces, or roughly 1½ shot glasses, of 80-proof spirits

12 ounces, or roughly one can or bottle, of beer

for keeping you alive longer by protecting your heart—as long as you practice moderation.

How Much to Drink

If you've been reading this chapter carefully, you'll notice that the exact amount of alcohol that you need to get a protective effect is not clear and varies from one study to another. This isn't all that surprising. Researchers can't measure every single factor in their subjects' lives, such as the amount of gin or wine taken in each glass. What's important to note is that the results all headed in exactly the same direction.

Alcohol is good for your cardiovascular health, but only in limited amounts. Just about every study finds a benefit from enjoying up to one to two drinks of alcohol daily. This coincides very nicely with the federal government's definition of moderate drinking, which is no more than one drink a day for women and no more than two for men.

But how much alcohol is in a drink?

When I was a medical student and could first afford to take my wife to a restaurant, I remember that a drink was much less substantial than the one you would get today. We drank from small wineglasses that were a little less than three-quarters filled. The spirits were measured in a 1-ounce jigger, and your drink normally contained just one jigger.

Today, the wine glasses are much larger and filled almost to the brim. And the bartender frequently does not hesitate to pour the spirits far beyond the 1-ounce limit.

As for beer, the quantity of beer by the bottle remains the same, but the glasses for draft beer, like the goblets for wine, have enlarged dramatically.

So how can you figure out exactly how much alcohol you need for sufficient protection against heart disease? In order to give you a feel for the amounts, let's use wine as a standard.

Wine. Wine is about 12 percent alcohol. So every 8 ounces of wine has 1 ounce of alcohol. Since your average wineglass holds about 6 ounces, a man needs one full glass of wine and one-third of a second glass. It is better that women drink one-half to two-thirds of this amount. A wineglass two-thirds full (4 ounces of wine) should do the cardiovascular trick.

Spirits. Because spirits such as vodka, scotch, and gin generally contain 40 percent alcohol, it will take only about one-third as much hard liquor as it does wine to deliver your daily dose of alcohol. For men, this means roughly 2.5 ounces. Women can cut this amount by a third to half; they need only about 1.5 ounces.

Beer. American beer is generally about 4 percent alcohol. At this concentration, it takes about three times as much beer as wine to give you your nutraceutical dose of alcohol. Assuming that a can of beer contains 12 ounces, that works out to 24 ounces, or two cans of beer a day. For women, that's a little more than a can or a bottle of beer daily.

If you don't like drinking alcohol, and these amounts make you feel sleepy or intoxicated, drink less. You may still enjoy the cardiac benefits at lower levels. The problem is that we do not know how much less. But if you have problems drinking the recommended volumes, just drink as much as you're comfortable with—up to that amount.

Here are a couple of thoughts to be sure that you get heart protection without raising your risk of harmful side effects or other diseases.

Spread out your dose. Apart from the other negative things that happen by drinking too much, the cardiac benefits of alcohol may disappear when you drink your entire week's supply at once. Alcohol metabolism doesn't work that way. Spread out your consumption through the week for maximum benefit.

Medication caution. Always talk to your doctor about possible interactions between alcohol and any drugs you may be taking, be they over-the-counter or prescription, such as painkillers, sedatives, and antihistamines.

Alcohol + Folic Acid = Potential Synergy

In chapter 9, I told you about some of the findings of Dr. Eric Rimm and his group at Harvard. Dr. Rimm has been following the health of more than 80,000 American women since 1976 as part of the Nurses' Health Study. He provided us with critical new evidence on the importance of folate and vitamin B_6 in the *Journal of the American Medical Association* in 1998.

Buried in the fine print of this study on the effects of the B vitamins was another intriguing finding. Dr. Rimm found that women who consumed the most folates and also drank one or more drinks of alcohol a day had a greater reduction of heart attacks than the other groups.

The women who were in the lowest folate-intake group but who consumed at least one drink a day were almost 20 percent less likely to experience heart disease than their sisters who took little folate and no booze.

In contrast, women who were in the group who took the most folate and who also consumed at least one drink daily were at 78 percent lower risk of coronary heart disease.

Let me put this impressive statistic another way: Women on a high-folate diet who also consumed more than one alcoholic beverage per day were about five times less at risk of heart disease than nondrinking women who didn't consume high amounts of folates.

These are impressive numbers indeed. The studies on men are ongoing, and the results will soon be published.

In the meantime, Dr. Rimm's findings are impressive because they offer good evidence that nutraceuticals—in this case, alcohol plus folic acid—can act together. But there's more to the story than that.

In this chapter, you have learned that a moderate consumption of alcohol can protect many of us from cardiovascular disease. I've touched on some of the reasons why men seem to be able to drink more than women for cardiac protection. Dr. Rimm's study provides important evidence that women who take folates may gain not only the same but even greater benefits than men do from alcohol alone. Look forward to further clinical studies on these exciting findings.

Are there reasons why the combination of alcohol and folates offers more protection for women than either of these nutraceuticals alone? One possibility is that these two nutraceuticals work to prevent heart disease through two clearly different mechanisms. The alcohol goes to work increasing women's HDL levels, slowing down their blood-clotting mechanisms, and so on. The folate attacks on the homocysteine front—and you'll recall from chapter 9 that homocysteine increases your risk of atherosclerosis.

Is Red Wine the Alcohol of Choice?

Red wine sales got a real boost in 1991 when an episode of the popular television show *60 Minutes* reported on what it called the French Paradox—the fact that the French are much less likely to die of heart disease than Americans despite their fat-laden diets. The French have one-third the incidence of heart attacks as Americans. The researchers attributed this effect to the fact that the consumption of wine in France is about 10 times that of North Americans.

Red wine's effectiveness as a heart disease preventative has been ascribed to the presence in red wine of substances called polyphenols. The term *polyphenol* is actually a catchall phrase that describes four different substances: flavonoids, soluble tannins, anthocyanins, and catechins. Some researchers think that polyphenols are particularly beneficial because the flavonoids in them are antioxidants. Just like vitamin E, the theory goes, flavonoids can neutralize free oxygen radicals in your blood vessels and prevent them from combining with your LDLs.

In theory, this makes sense. But as of now, there's no convincing clinical evidence to suggest that red wine offers any advantage over other forms of liquor in protecting against heart disease. The active ingredient in all liquor is ethanol. It's in red wine, white wine, beer, vodka, gin, and every other alcoholic beverage.

In an intriguing animal study in 1996, researchers led by Benvenuto Cestaro, Ph.D., of the department of medical chemistry and biochemistry at Università degli Studi di Milano in Italy, fed rats either pure ethanol, red wine, or wine from which the ethanol had been removed, then tested the animals' blood for its antioxidant properties. The upshot was that none of the positive effects of red wine were tracked to the polyphenols. When the researchers separated red wine into its two components, the protective ability went with the alcohol, not with the polyphenols. Blood from the ethanol-fed and wine-fed animals showed much stronger antioxidant properties than the blood containing just the nonalcoholic polyphenols. In addition, the researchers found that animals receiving alcohol had the highest levels of internally synthesized vitamin E. Maybe these nutraceuticals were working together—another possible example of an effective nutraceutical combination.

Dr. Rimm and a team of researchers from the department of nutrition at the Harvard School of Public Health and the Kaiser Permanente Medical Center and the Division of Research Group in Oakland, California, produced an important paper in 1996. It systematically reviewed every single study available after 1965 that provided specific information on consumption of beer, wine, or spirits in relation to risk of coronary heart disease. In the end, Dr. Rimm concluded that all alcoholic drinks are linked with lower risk. His group found no advantage to one source of alcohol over another.

Beer, spirits, and wines of different types can prevent heart disease and also reduce the incidence of heart attacks and strokes. No single alcoholic substance has demonstrated superiority. It is primarily alcohol that does the job.

Should You Start Drinking If You're an Abstainer?

The American Heart Association says that the answer to this question is no. But I think that my distinguished colleagues and even the usually enthusiastic mass media have become overly cautious when it comes to recommending alcohol. They are hesitant to deliver the truth about alcohol's important cardiac protection. I don't think that they argue with the medical evidence that demonstrates alcohol's protective effect. Rather, I think that they're justifiably concerned about the risks associated with alcohol abuse.

I understand their concern. The costs of alcohol abuse are staggering, both in dollars and in suffering. And if you have any reason to believe that you won't be able to control your drinking if you start, then I would advise against using alcohol as a nutraceutical. But since the clinical results of studies on behalf of this one of nature's medicines is so compelling, I can't help thinking that the excessive reluctance to recommend alcohol comes in part from a little bit of Puritanism. Taking a drink still has a taint of immorality and licentiousness about it.

Here's the plain truth: Those who totally abstain from alcohol are more likely to suffer heart disease and heart attacks than those who drink. Many people use alcohol safely and so protect their hearts from the pathology that leads to heart disease.

The decision of whether to drink or not to drink is yours to make. If drinking alcohol conflicts with your religious or moral beliefs, if you have alcoholism in your family or a tendency to drink too much, or if you suffer from congestive heart failure, don't use it. I urge you to discuss this issue with your doctor.

PART THREE

Beyond
Carnitine

CHAPTER TWELVE

Nature's Cholesterol Controllers

At many places in this book, I have urged you to get beyond an unhealthy preoccupation with cholesterol. I have emphasized that the best strategy for preventing heart disease is a multipronged approach that tries to prevent each of the pathologic processes that contribute to heart disease.

For purposes of this chapter, forget what I said. Let's talk about cholesterol. Though controlling it is not the single answer to preventing heart disease, your cholesterol level is important. While it's true that many people who have heart disease don't have elevated cholesterol, it's also true that normal is better than high. As a rule of thumb, experts say that for every 1 percent decrease in your total cholesterol, you get a 2 percent decrease in your risk of heart disease. So, theoretically, if you can cut your cholesterol from 250 milligrams per deciliter (mg/dl) to 200 mg/dl, you could reduce your risk of heart disease by 40 percent. I say "theoretically" because the cholesterol guidelines recommended by experts are just that—

Cholesterol Levels: How High Is High According to the Experts?

There is some disagreement about exactly what levels of cholesterol put you at special risk for developing heart disease. Many experts use guidelines from the National Cholesterol Education Program (NCEP).

Remember, there are two types of cholesterol: LDL, or low-density lipoprotein, which is bad for you, and HDL, or high-density lipoprotein, which is actually good for you. Keep in mind that your ratio of LDL to HDL is a very important number. Most experts agree that your LDL should be no more than 3.5 times your HDL. The higher it goes over that, the greater your risk of heart disease.

The NCEP guidelines indicate desirable levels as total blood cholesterol of less than 200 milligrams per deciliter (mg/dl), LDL cholesterol of lower than 130 mg/dl, and HDL cholesterol of higher than 60 mg/dl.

guidelines, based on averages rather than on individual differences. And these numbers are only estimates, which could change as we learn more.

It's important to understand that much of your cholesterol is manufactured by your body in your liver. Your dietary intake of cholesterol accounts for a smaller but significant fraction of your total cholesterol level than what your liver produces. So, despite all the publicity about the importance of lowering your cholesterol by limiting the fat and cholesterol in your diet, for many people, dietary restrictions may not help you. Plenty of folks can go on pretty strict diets and find their total cholesterol reduced only slightly. Indeed, in the most extreme cases, some people eat virtually no fat or cholesterol and yet can't get their cholesterol levels down at all.

There are some drug options (see "The Six Statins," on page 202). There's no question that we have powerful pharmaceuticals available today that can lower your cholesterol level. But we've been able to evaluate the statin drugs for only about five years, and they may have long-term side effects that haven't cropped up yet. It's definitely worth the risk of taking such drugs if your cholesterol is 260 mg/dl or higher and you can't lower it by any other means. But I don't think that you should be chancing drugs if your cholesterol is normal or even at the top end of normal, in other words, up to 250 mg/dl or so. Why not consider trying some nutraceutical options before going the pharmaceutical route?

This chapter includes a few substances that may help lower cholesterol. Though I don't think that the clinical evidence is strong enough to include these nutraceuticals as part of the Cardiac Elixir, there are some indications that these natural substances can be safe, natural alternatives or additions to cholesterol-lowering medications. As always, I suggest you consult with your physician before taking any of these products.

Plant Stanol Esters

If this doesn't ring a bell, it's because stanol esters have yet to take off in a big way in the United States. That's not the case elsewhere in the world. Much of the research on these substances has been done in Finland since the early 1990s; more than one million people in Finland have used this product safely since 1995. In fact, about 20 percent of all households in Finland use a margarine substitute called Benecol, which contains plant stanol esters, to lower their overall cholesterol and low-density lipoprotein (LDL) levels.

What it is: Plant stanols and sterols belong to what's known as the phytosterol family of compounds. Basically, they're the plant equivalent of cholesterol. They are found in small quantities in many plant and vegetable oils, including oils extracted from pine trees, soy, beans, rice, corn, and wheat. The plant stanols in Benecol are an extract of pine bark, while those in Take Control, another margarine substitute on the market in the United States, contain sterols and come from soybean oil. If you eat vegetable oils and margarines, you may be getting as much as 160 to 360 milligrams of sterols daily, plus

A Profile of Plant Stanol Esters

What they are:
Plant extracts

What they do:
Lower your overall cholesterol level by 10 percent on average and "bad" low-density lipoprotein (LDL) cholesterol levels by 14 percent

Mechanism of protection:
May reduce your risk of coronary artery disease

Where you can buy it:
In pharmacies and supermarkets

What to look for on the label:
Contains plant stanol esters or plant sterol esters; products now on the market in the United States include Benecol, a patented margarine-like substance containing plant stanol esters, and Take Control, another patented spread containing plant sterol esters.

Who it's for:
Anyone over the age of 35 with high levels of cholesterol or high normal LDL levels (levels of 220 to 240 milligrams per deciliter)

How much to take:
2 to 3 grams daily, which works out to 2 to 3 pats of Benecol or Take Control margarine substitute daily.

another 20 to 50 milligrams of stanols. That adds up to around a third of a gram of these substances in your diet—not enough to have a measurable effect on cutting your cholesterol. As you can see in "A Profile of Plant Stanol Esters," you need 2 to 3 grams daily.

At the Foundation for Innovation in Medicine (FIM) conference on nutraceuticals and pharmaceuticals in November 1998, Nilo Cater, M.D., a leader in the field of lipid research at the Center for Human Nutrition in Dallas, summarized the results of some 100 papers on these substances that appeared between 1950 and 1976. In total, these studies evaluated the effects of plant stanols and sterols on more than 1,800 subjects. Some studies showed that they could lower cholesterol levels by 10 to 20 percent. These studies provided people with stanols and sterols via a variety of formulations: granules, liquids, powders, tablets, and capsules. The results tended to vary depending on what type of formulation was used. In addition, people had to take very high amounts of these substances for the cholesterol-lowering effect to kick in.

By the mid-1970s, Scott Grundy, M.D., Ph.D., of the Center for Human Nutrition at the University of Texas Southwestern Medical Center in Dallas, a pioneer in this field, began to evaluate the effectiveness of much smaller amounts of these substances. At first, Dr. Grundy and his researchers found that 3 grams daily of the sterols were just as effective as higher amounts. At the same time, other researchers exploring the possibilities of this family of natural substances discovered that stanols were even more effective than sterols.

But the effect of both substances on LDL cholesterol varied, depending on whether the researchers used capsules, pills, or other formulations of stanols. The scientific breakthrough—a substance that people could take in relatively small amounts and get reliable results—came when the Raiso Company, a pharmaceutical firm in Finland, came up with a process called esterification. This process converts plant stanol into a fat-soluble substance called a plant stanol ester. In this physical state, the plant stanol dissolves well into fatty foods, such as margarines or salad dressings. Plant stanol ester is colorless and tasteless, but once dissolved in these edible fats, it seems to be reliable and effective at lowering cholesterol.

What it does: Plant phytosterol and stanol molecules are almost identical structurally to the cholesterol in your body. Basically, your digestive tract can't tell the difference between these molecules and cholesterol. What this means is that when plant stanols get to your intestines, they look so much like cholesterol to your body that they compete with cholesterol for absorption. Simply put, your body is tricked by the stanol esters into absorbing less cholesterol because the presence of plant stanol esters interferes with the absorption of real cholesterols from your intestine. As a result, less cholesterol returns to your liver, so your liver works harder to synthesize more cholesterol. It increases its uptake of the cholesterol that's in your blood and also processes more LDL, which results in a drop in your LDL (bad) cholesterol level. The result? Stanol esters in your intestinal tract translate into lower total cholesterol and LDL levels in your blood.

Many randomized double-blind clinical trials published in respected scientific journals report that 2 to 3 grams of plant stanol esters daily (which translates into three pats of margarine or the equivalent) will reduce your LDL cholesterol level by 10 to 20 percent. Plant stanol esters were reported to be effective among healthy men and women, people who have just had heart attacks, and people with type 2 (adult-onset) diabetes.

I'd like to sum up just two of these reports.

The landmark study was published in the November 1995 issue of the *New England Journal of Medicine* by Tatu A. Miettinen, M.D., and others in the department of medicine at the University of Helsinki in Finland. One hundred and fifty-three otherwise healthy people in Finland who had mildly elevated levels of cholesterol in their blood used either ordinary margarine spread for a year or margarine with plant stanol ester. The group using ordinary margarine showed no changes in their total cholesterol levels. The group that used the stanol ester spread experienced a 10 percent reduction in their overall cholesterol levels and a 14 percent reduction in their LDL cholesterol levels. Then, the subjects discontinued using both these spreads. Two months later, the investigators remeasured everyone's cholesterol levels. The group that had used ordinary margarine maintained the same cholesterol levels as before, but the group that had been using stanol esters went back to where they had started—proof that the stanol ester was responsible for their lower cholesterol levels.

Another two-part study, published in *Circulation* in 1997 and led by Helena Gylling, M.D., of the Department of Medicine in the Division of Internal Medicine at the University of Helsinki, first followed the cholesterol levels of 22 postmenopausal women in Finland for 7 weeks. The women were divided into three groups. One group ate a low-fat, low-cholesterol diet at home following dieticians' suggestions, the second group ate three servings daily of rapeseed oil margarine or canola oil margarine, and the third used the plant stanol ester spread Benecol. The margarine group experienced a 4 to 5 percent reduction of total and

LDL cholesterol over the low-fat, low-cholesterol home diet group, while the plant stanol ester group had an additional 14 to 15 percent reduction in LDL cholesterol over what the individuals on the canola diet had achieved. This effect was achieved within 7 weeks.

For the second part of this study, the researchers went on to look at the effects of stanol ester margarine on the cholesterol levels of 10 women who were already taking a medication called simvastatin to lower their cholesterol levels. Simvastatin belongs to a group of drugs called statins. These drugs reduce the amount of cholesterol that the liver can produce, which also encourages the liver to pick up cholesterol from the blood, thus lowering cholesterol levels.

As I just pointed out, stanol esters reduce cholesterol through a different mechanism. They work in the intestine to reduce your absorption of intestinal cholesterol, so they should be able to lower cholesterol above and beyond what statins can do. And there's evidence that this can happen. In the study I just mentioned, the women on medication alone experienced about a 35 percent reduction of their LDL cholesterol levels. That was an expected result, based on the results of many previous studies. What is impressive is that when they incorporated three servings of the Benecol plant stanol ester spread into their diets, there was an additional 14 to 16 percent reduction in their LDL levels after 12 weeks. This presents the possibility that plant stanol esters can effectively lower cholesterol beyond the levels of conventional medications when added to them—a good example of the potential benefits of nutraceuticals and pharmaceuticals working together.

Tu Nguyen, M.D., cholesterol director at the Mayo Clinic in Rochester, Minnesota, is evaluating a study into the effects of Benecol on blood cholesterol levels, and preliminary results point to the same 14 percent reduction in LDL levels. Though the evidence for plant sterols (the substance available in Take Control) is not quite as strong, there has been one major study that indicates that plant sterols can be just as effective at lowering your

The Six Statins

The six statins are a family of powerful cholesterol-lowering drugs: lovastatin (sold under the brand name Mevacor), fluvastatin (Lescol), pravastatin (Pravachol), simvastatin (Zocor), cervastatin (Baycol), and atorvastatin (Lipitor). These drugs work by interfering with the capacity of the liver to make cholesterol and by increasing the liver's ability to remove cholesterol from the bloodstream. In addition to lowering total cholesterol levels, the statins can reduce LDL levels by up to 60 percent.

It's also clear that over a 5-year period, the statins that have been studied significantly lower your risk of dying from a heart attack. But here's the big uncertainty about the statin drugs: Because they are reasonably new on the scene, we just don't have data on what happens to people who take these medications for 10 to 30 years. These are very powerful pharmaceuticals that affect a fundamental metabolic process.

That's why I'm troubled by one development: the effort to promote the use of these drugs even among people with normal or high-end-of-normal cholesterol levels. Though lower cholesterol is generally better than high cholesterol, unless your cholesterol is above 240 milligrams per deciliter (mg/dl), I would recommend using the Cardiac Elixir and substances such as Benecol or Take Control before you start on drugs.

cholesterol levels. Unlike plant stanols, though, plant sterols are absorbed, and the long-term effects of this have not been evaluated.

Red Rice Yeast

Thousands of people in Asia may have a health secret that we can share. In one form or another, a substance called red rice yeast has been a staple in the occidental diet for centuries. It's not yet known whether these ingested amounts have had a significant impact on reducing heart disease, but a growing body of

What about borderline-high cholesterol levels? Many expert physicians think that once your cholesterol level exceeds 240 mg/dl (or even lower), your condition is dangerous to your health and should be treated with statins or other cholesterol-lowering drugs. But I am not convinced that the line between healthy and dangerous is that clear-cut. Cholesterol ranges are based on epidemiological data, a fancy way of describing statistical averages of large populations. There is a large "gray zone" where, in my opinion, taking the Cardiac Elixir rather than drugs makes a lot of sense.

So my view is this: Don't go right to the statins as a quick cholesterol fix. Try nutraceuticals—both the ingredients in the Cardiac Elixir and the substances in this chapter. You may be able to lower your cholesterol 10 percent from the borderline-high zone of 220 to 240 mg/dl with these natural substances. If they don't get your cholesterol down to where it belongs, talk to your doctor about whether statins are right for you. Of course, if your physician believes that your cholesterol is unacceptably high and puts you on statins, he or she is doing the right thing. It's worth taking on the risk of pharmaceuticals. I would strongly recommend, however, that you take the Cardiac Elixir along with your cholesterol-lowering drugs.

evidence indicates that red rice yeast may be able to lower your cholesterol.

What it is: Red rice yeast (called *Hung-chu* or *Hong Qu* in Chinese) is one of the by-products of rice fermentation. It's a yeast produced by several different types of *Monascus* fungi that grow on and in the rice. In China, the red yeast is usually prepared by mixing red wine mash, natural juice of *Polygonum* grass, and alum water with rice. The natural fermentation product has been used for some 2,000 years in China for making rice wine, as a food preservative, and as a digestive aid. Red yeast's medical potential first came to light in an ancient Chinese pharmacy book published during the Ming Dynasty called *Ben Cao Gang Mu–Dan Shi Bu Yi*. It was described as a mild, nonpoisonous substance, good for treating indigestion, diarrhea, and problems with blood circulation, the spleen, and the stomach.

In 1977, Professor Akira Endo, in Japan, discovered that a strain of this yeast could produce substances that block the metabolic pathway for cholesterol production by the liver. Researchers took over from there to refine and test the product on animals and people.

The reported clinical data are positive. Studies around the world—in animals and in humans—show that this yeast seems to lower cholesterol without reported toxicity. Red rice yeast is not easy to come by. It's most readily available in a patented product called Cholestin, which was developed by a company called Pharmanex and is now marketed by NuSkin. Seventeen independent trials in China alone, providing 872 patients with 0.6 to 2.4 grams of Cholestin daily for 8 weeks, reported that this substance reduced the total serum cholesterol of the subjects by 11.2 to 32.2 percent.

Here in the United States, David Heber, M.D., Ph.D., director of the University of California, Los Angeles, Center for Human Nutrition, ran a double-blind randomized clinical trial of red rice yeast on 83 healthy people whose cholesterol was at the high end of normal or low end of high (on average, about 250 milligrams per deciliter). The subjects took either a placebo or 2.4 grams of the red rice yeast in the form of Cholestin for 8 weeks. Those who took this nutraceutical cut total cholesterol levels by 18 percent and their LDL levels by 23 percent.

What it does: Red yeast works by blocking the enzyme that your liver uses to make cholesterol. Since your liver makes about 80 percent of your body's cholesterol, this action can effectively reduce your body's overall blood cholesterol levels. Cholestin contains at least 10 different substances that actively inhibit this enzyme, plus unsaturated fatty acids, which may lower triglyceride levels and increase levels of high-density lipoproteins (HDLs)—the "good" cholesterol.

Red rice yeast is controversial. Ronald Krauss, M.D., chairman of the American Heart Association's nutrition committee, is concerned about use of Cholestin. The chemical structure of one of red rice yeast's dozen or so active ingredients is a substance called mevinolin, which is remarkably similar to the FDA-approved synthetic drug lovastatin. And lovastatin is the active pharmaceutical ingredient of Mevacor, one of a family of effective medications prescribed by doctors to lower high cholesterol. Dr. Krauss fears that people who should be on prescription drugs will choose to take red yeast instead—without physician supervision.

I share these concerns. That's why I have constantly reminded you to check with your doctor before taking nutraceuticals.

Candidates for Cholestin are people over the age of 35 with high cholesterol levels. The recommended dose, based on studies in China and the United States, is 4 capsules daily (there are 600 milligrams of red rice yeast per capsule). Some people might experience heartburn or other mild digestive upset. It's available in selected pharmacies, supermarkets, and Chinese medicine stores. Cholestin is also sold, like Tupperware, through multilevel marketing in private homes.

Niacin

For almost half a century, we've seen data to suggest that niacin can reduce your "bad" LDL cholesterol levels by 10 to 20 percent, reduce your triglycerides—another type of fat particle found in the blood of healthy people and in elevated amounts in people with diabetes and people with certain genetic diseases—by 20 to 50 percent, and raise your levels of "good" HDL cholesterol by 15 to 35 percent.

What it is: Niacin, also known as nicotinic acid or vitamin B_3, is a water-soluble vitamin that plays many crucial metabolic roles. The best food sources of niacin in food are liver and organ meats, eggs, fish, brewer's yeast, rice bran, wheat bran, and peanuts, though you can get some of this nutrient in unprocessed rice and other grains, some nuts, and legumes. Some researchers even feel that niacin is at least as effective as today's newer lipid-lowering drugs.

One study compared the effects of niacin and lovastatin (a member of the statin cholesterol-lowering drug family) on 136 patients at five different lipid clinics.

After 26 weeks, lovastatin did lower bad LDL cholesterol levels more (32 percent compared with 23 percent). But when it came to raising the good HDL cholesterol, niacin was far more effective (33 percent) than lovastatin (7 percent). Niacin also lowered a fat called Lp(a) lipoprotein, which is similar in structure to LDL and also a risk factor for heart disease, by 35 percent. Lovastatin had no effect on this blood fat.

In yet another study, gemfibrozil (a lipid-lowering drug) increased HDL by only 10 percent, lovastatin increased HDL by only 6 percent, while niacin bumped it by a very respectable 30 percent. In fact, a 1986 article published in the *Journal of the American Medical Association* recommended that doctors suggest niacin as the first "drug" that people should take if a low-fat diet alone fails to lower high cholesterol levels.

What it does: Niacin is an important component of a number of enzymes, including those responsible for energy production; fat, cholesterol, and carbohydrate metabolism; and the manufacture of many body compounds and hormones. Niacin decreases the production of triglycerides in your liver. And since your body eventually converts triglycerides into LDLs, taking niacin encourages the level of this lipid to fall as well.

Niacin may also reduce your fibrinogen levels, which makes your platelets less sticky. If true, niacin could reduce the opportunity for clot formation in your arteries, which could lower your odds of plaque formation, blockages, and even heart attacks. One landmark study of 8,000 middle-aged men who had suffered one heart attack has indicated that niacin taken after a heart attack may help you live longer. Another study, the Coronary Drug Project, reported that men who took at least 2 grams of niacin daily for 5 years suffered significantly less heart disease than those treated with a placebo. Even 10 niacin-free years after the end of the study, the group that had taken niacin for 5 years had 20 percent fewer manifestations of heart disease.

You probably ingest about 15 to 35 milligrams of niacin daily, but that's not enough to make any measurable dent on your blood lipid levels. You need about 1.5 to 3 grams daily to lower your blood lipid levels.

Now, here's a caution: The biggest reason why niacin is not a core component of my Cardiac Elixir is that in some people, niacin supplements have side effects that range from annoying to dangerous. The most common is an immediate skin flushing and/or itchiness for up to 45 minutes. This is usually harmless. It's caused by niacin's effect on your arteries and the nerves that regulate them.

Other side effects could include high levels of uric acid in your blood (which could cause arthritis-like pain in your joints), abnormalities in liver function, and excess blood sugar. These effects will usually disappear when you stop taking niacin. On top of this, niacin may have other worrisome side effects on your body organs, your liver in particular. These could include nausea, jaundice, or even elevated liver enzymes. Very rarely, vitamin B_3 could also cause blurry vision or skin discoloration in the armpits or groin.

In addition, nicotinic acid at the dose necessary to improve serum lipids can make the diabetes more difficult to control. It's especially important that you talk to your doctor before taking niacin supplements.

An alternative form of vitamin B_3, called flush–free or inositol-bound niacin, also known as inositol hexaniacinate, has become available in the United States. As I write this, I am not familiar with this preparation, but I do know that this form of the vitamin has been used in Europe for decades and reportedly does not cause any toxic side effects. Don't assume this form will prevent the flushing and itching, but talk to your doctor about trying it.

Sometimes, taking sustained-release capsules, which release nicotinic acid gradually from your stomach into your blood instead of all at once, can help you avoid flushing and itching. But for some people, that kind of capsule can have even more toxic side effects. One study published in the *Journal of the American Medical Association* reported that an alarming 52 percent of patients taking sustained-release niacin developed liver damage and that 78 percent of patients stopped taking sustained-release niacin because of side effects.

In many people, niacin supplements can help control cholesterol. But because of the possible side effects, it should be taken only under a doctor's care. Even if your doctor recommends it, he may suggest that you get a liver function test every few months to be sure that it's not doing any damage. (Incidentally, many of the drugs to lower cholesterol require the same kind of monitoring.) You should definitely *not* supplement with niacin if you have had any problems with your liver or gallbladder, if you have gout, if you have diabetes (niacin may increase blood sugar levels or impair glucose tolerance), or if you're pregnant.

Let there be no doubt that niacin is a fascinating substance that urgently needs more clinical research to better define who should take it.

Soy

What it is: Soy is a combination of substances, including natural amino acids and isoflavones, found in soybeans.

In November 1998, the FDA issued an important ruling. It officially decreed that companies selling foods containing soy protein could claim that this substance may lower heart disease risk by reducing blood levels of total cholesterol and "bad" LDL cholesterol. The good news is that there is plenty of evidence that soy can be a cholesterol cutter. The bad news is that it doesn't appear to cut cholesterol very much. On the other hand, it may have beneficial effects beyond lowering cholesterol.

After reviewing every single published human clinical trial available to date, the FDA acknowledged that consumption of 25 grams of soy protein per day on a long-term basis (up to a year) could lower your serum cholesterol level by at least 4 percent. Of the 46 studies reviewed by the FDA, 91 percent reported a decrease in total cholesterol; of the 41 studies that reported on "bad" LDL cholesterol, 98 percent reported a decrease; and of the 39 that measured "good" HDL cholesterol, 97 percent reported either no change or increases.

Foods High in Soy

To enjoy the full cardiovascular benefits of soy, you need both its protein and its isoflavonoids. Soybeans that have been hulled, flaked, or defatted may have full protein content, but they are probably low in isoflavonoids. Good food sources of soy protein include miso, soybeans, soy bran, soy flour, soy grits or meal, soy milk, soy nuts, soy sauce, soy yogurt, tempeh (a textured soy protein), and tofu.

Only in America are the health benefits of soy considered news. A central component of the diet in many Asian countries for millenia (its first recorded use is in the *Materia Medica* of the Chinese Emperor Shen Nung in 2838 B.C.), soy comes from soybeans—a member of the legume family. Buddhist missionaries took tofu, a curdlike product extracted from soybeans, from China to Japan and Korea between the second and seventh centuries. It's inexpensive, rich in fiber, and provides a complete protein just as useful to the body as the protein in meat, cheese, or eggs.

The clinical data on soy's effectiveness are rather impressive. To begin with, many studies show that countries like Japan and China, where soy is an integral component of the daily diet, also have lower rates of heart disease than the United States. More scientific evidence of soy's ability to reduce heart disease in animals first cropped up in the early part of the twentieth century and has grown since. The first of many studies suggesting that soy might be able to lower cholesterol in humans appeared in 1967. Almost three decades of research later, in 1995, a team led by James Anderson, M.D., director of the University of Kentucky Health Management Resources Weight Management program and chief of the endocrine-metabolic section at the Veterans Affairs Medical Center in Lexington, came up with results that the medical community took seriously.

Dr. Anderson's landmark study ran in the respected *New England Journal of Medicine*. It was what's called a meta-analysis. He and his team reviewed and analyzed 38 previous studies—just about every one conducted until that point—involving 730 people who had high cholesterol levels. Here's what they found.

Overall, people who ate an average of 47 grams of soy protein daily in the form of soy milk, soy protein, and tofu enjoyed a 9 percent reduction in total cholesterol, a 13 percent reduction in LDL cholesterol, an 11 percent reduction in triglycerides, and a 2 percent increase in HDL cholesterol. The people with the highest initial cholesterol levels showed the greatest overall serum cholesterol reductions (24 percent) when they substituted soy products for red meat.

Dr. Anderson concluded that soy protein can measurably cut down on the amount of cholesterol, LDL cholesterol, and triglyercides in your blood.

Subsequent research has revealed that soy seems to be good for you whether or not you have high cholesterol. A study published in the *American Journal of Clinical Nutrition* in 1998 demonstrated this quite nicely. It examined the effect of substituting soy protein for animal protein on 26 men. The subjects all ate according to what's called the National Cholesterol Educational Program Step I diet—the low-fat diet that most doctors recommend to people as a first step in lowering blood cholesterol. Half of the men had normal levels of cholesterol, while the other half had high (above 250 milligrams per deciliter) cholesterol. The soy protein diet significantly lowered the LDL levels and the ratio of LDL to HDL in both groups of men. The soy protein was effective above and beyond an accepted standard dietary regimen.

What it does: Skeptics might suggest that soy may be good for your heart simply because it replaces high-fat foods like meats. Indeed, the Anderson study reported that the more you substitute soy for meat, the more it seems to lower your cholesterol level. But researchers are finding that the protein component of soy protein, unlike protein from animal and most other vegetable proteins, appears to alter the synthesis and metabolism of cholesterol in the liver. It may enhance bile acid secretion, and bile effectively removes cholesterol from the blood.

What's probably more important, and a considerable body of research is building to support this, is that soy's unique plant hormones—a class of substances called isoflavones—are the secret of its effectiveness. These substances appear to latch on to the same receptors on cells as estrogen, a potent natural heart protector for women during their fertile years. They seem to provide protection very similar to that provided by estrogen.

Studies on monkeys, hamsters, rabbits, rats, and yes, humans, have corroborated the ability of isoflavonoids to act independently of soy proteins on blood cholesterol concentrations. In one important study, monkeys that were fed soy protein without isoflavones showed no change in their blood lipid levels; when fed diets rich in isoflavones, their overall cholesterol levels dropped. Not only that, the monkeys that ate soy protein plus isoflavones had significantly less atherosclerosis.

Overall, the isoflavones in soy (in combination with its protein) appear to do one or all of the following:

■ *Lower overall cholesterol levels by 7 to 10 percent and LDL levels by somewhat more; many studies have consistently demonstrated this effect.*

■ *Act as antioxidants; laboratory studies show that isoflavones tend to scavenge free oxygen radicals from your blood, thus preventing these volatile molecules from combining with LDL cholesterol molecules and turning into plaque.*

■ *Help slow down blood clotting and thus reduce the likelihood of atherosclerosis or a blocked artery; they seem to act on one of the enzymes that tells your platelets to clump together.*

■ *Stimulate cells in your arteries' walls to produce nitric acid, a natural vasodilator that encourages the vessel to stay open and relaxed when needed.*

■ *Keep artery walls more elastic; one study among 221 menopausal and perimenopausal women found that it was just as effective as estrogen.*

■ *Inhibit the growth of the smooth muscle cells that are part of the atherosclerosis process; this effect has been demonstrated in the laboratory so far, not in people.*

Soy is a good dietary idea for everybody over age 35. It's perfectly safe, is one of the oldest foods known to man, and has been a staple in Asian diets for centuries. Postmenopausal women, in particular, would do well to add soy to their diets. You can buy foods containing soy in supermarkets, health food stores, and other retail outlets. I suggest that you aim for around 25 grams daily, 30 grams if you have heart disease.

If you don't want to eat soy foods regularly, you can get the benefit by supplementing with a couple of spoonfuls of soy protein powder daily. Some people put soy powder in fruit shakes.

Fiber

Americans have been interested in fiber ever since the 1830s, when Sylvester Graham created the Graham cracker and successfully marketed it as a cure-all for the nation's health problems. Fiber may protect your heart health by lowering your cholesterol level.

What it is: Fiber is the part of a plant that is not digested by our enzymes. There are two main types of fiber. Insoluble fiber, the kind that does not dissolve in water, provides roughage in the form of bulk, which your digestive system needs to stay in good order. Found in wheat bran, lima beans, peanuts, seeds, and many legumes, fruits, and vegetables, this type of fiber doesn't do much for your heart. It may have a kind of secondary protective effect in that it tends to be filling so that you may be able to resist the temptation to eat too much fat. But at the moment, there is no direct evidence that insoluble fiber enhances your heart health.

On the other hand, water-soluble fiber, a type that dissolves in water, seems to be a cholesterol fighter. This is the type of fiber found in grains such as oat bran, barley, psyllium, legumes, some vegetables, and some fruits.

What it does: Water-soluble fiber appears to work by binding with bile acids, which contain cholesterol (as well as many other substances) and also function to help your body absorb and digest fats, including cholesterol. It may also increase the amount of bile

Good Food Sources of Soluble Fiber

These sources of soluble fiber are a tasty way of lowering your risk of heart disease.

• Apples	• Oat flour
• Barley	• Oatmeal
• Beans, baked	• Oats, whole
• Beans, white	• Peas, dried
• Guar gum	• Prunes
• Lentils	• Rice bran
• Oat bran	• Strawberries

acid that your body produces. The upshot is that the soluble fiber you eat turns bile acids and cholesterol into a gel-like mass that surrounds food particles in your small intestine. Once your body has excreted this mass, you're left with low levels of bile acids circulating in your blood. That's a signal to your liver that it needs to convert cholesterol into more bile acid, which then binds with more soluble fiber and is excreted. In other words, the process perpetuates itself. Soluble fibers may also change how your liver handles cholesterol. And they may alter how quickly you digest or absorb certain lipids in the first place.

The evidence on behalf of fiber began emerging long ago. As far back as the 1960s, two researchers, Denis Burkitt, M.D., and Hugh Trowell, compared disease rates and dietary factors between Africa and North America. They pointed out that there might be a connection between the high level of unrefined plant food in the African diet and the rarity of heart disease there. By 1988, the Surgeon General's Report on Nutrition and Health pointed out that soluble fibers, such as pectins or gums, seemed to reduce cholesterol levels by 10 to 15 percent. The very next year, in 1989, the National Research Council's volume on diet and health pointed out that soluble fibers such as pectin, guar gum, or oat bran can significantly reduce total cholesterol and LDL levels.

A Fiber Caution

If you suddenly increase the amount of fiber in your diet, regardless of the source, you may experience constipation or cramps. That's because soluble fiber must dissolve in water to keep it from becoming dry and constipating. So drink six to eight 8-ounce glasses of water throughout the day. In addition, some high-fiber foods can stimulate the formation of intestinal gases, which can make you feel bloated and flatulent until your system adjusts. To avoid this, increase your fiber intake gradually. You can also use substances available on the market, such as Beano, which can reduce flatulence.

Finally, in 1998, the FDA conducted a review of all the scientific evidence available for the health benefits of the soluble fiber found in psyllium and oat bran. It evaluated more than 55 studies conducted over three decades linking psyllium to cholesterol levels and found that 52 of them showed a reduction in cholesterol levels. Overall, researchers found that as little as 2.5 grams daily in one study could reduce cholesterol levels, though as much as 30 grams daily in another was equally beneficial.

The cholesterol-cutting effect was pretty much universal—among people with normal cholesterol and people with high cholesterol, among men and women, and among adults and children—whether they took fiber for periods as short as 9 days or over a sustained period of as long as 29 months. The FDA also reviewed 33 studies investigating the effect of oat bran on heart health. Twenty-two reported a reduction in cholesterol levels.

To be more specific:

■ *Two studies published in the* Journal of the American College of Nutrition *provide good clinical evidence. In one, the researchers supplemented the diets of 23 people with oat fiber extract for a mere 5 weeks and found that their total and LDL cholesterol levels both dropped significantly. Another, published just last year, looked at the cholesterol levels of 66 men ages 20 to 45 who added cookies fortified with 2.6 grams of the soluble fibers oat bran or psyllium to their reduced-fat diets. Within 8 weeks, their LDL cholesterol levels were down by 23 to 26 percent. A control group of men who ate cookies made with wheat bran (containing insoluble fiber instead of soluble fiber) also experienced a drop in LDL levels, but it was much more modest—only 8 percent.*

■ *A double-blind study among 248 people conducted by James Anderson, M.D., professor of medicine at the University of Kentucky College of Medicine in Lexington, and his colleagues found that people who had mild to moderately elevated levels of cholesterol could reduce their blood cholesterol levels by an average of 8.6 percent and LDL levels by 11.1 percent within 6 months (compared with 4 percent reductions for the group given a placebo) by sticking to a low-fat diet and eating psyllium twice daily. The psyllium worked best for the people with the highest cholesterol levels, reducing them by up to 25 percent.*

■ *Another study published in* Nutrition Research *found that even 2 weeks on a high-fiber diet (mostly leafy vegetables, fruit, and nuts) was enough to bring cholesterol levels down by more than 20 percent and LDL levels down just as substantially.*

■ *Yet another report—a meta-analysis of 11 published and unpublished studies of 404 subjects who ate 7 to 12 grams daily of soluble fiber in psyllium-enriched breakfast cereal—reported that the fiber lowered overall blood cholesterol levels by 5 percent and LDL levels by 9 percent.*

■ *In 1996, the Health Professionals Follow-Up Study, which assessed the health and diet of thousands of men for 6 years, reported that the more vegetable, fruit, and cereal fiber the men ate, the lower their risk of having a heart attack. Cereal fiber was the most effective at reducing heart attack risk.*

■ *As for women, the June 1999 issue of the* Journal of the American Medical Association *reported similar findings among the thousands of female participants in the Nurses' Health Study. Overall, the higher their intake—cereals showed the strongest protective effect—the lower their risk of coronary heart disease.*

■ *The Iowa Women's Health Study, which studied more than 34,000 healthy postmenopausal women between 1986 and 1995, found that the more whole-grain products they ate, the lower their risk of heart disease. It defined a diet appropriately high in whole grains as 1.9 to 3.2 servings of whole grains daily.*

■ *The study you read about in chapter 8 on male smokers that showed an effect of small doses of vitamin E on their heart health also demonstrated the benefits of fiber. When the smoking middle-aged Finnish men in this study increased their dietary fiber by 10 grams (about three slices of rye bread), their risk of coronary death dropped by as much as 17 percent. The benefit was even stronger (31 percent less risk of a heart attack) after adjusting for other dietary factors, such as beta-carotene, vitamins C and E, alcohol, and saturated fatty acids.*

Taken all together, this body of evidence is compelling. But some still-skeptical researchers point out that it might be other substances in high-fiber foods—such as phytochemicals, antioxidants, minerals, phytoestrogens, or vitamins—that confer heart protection, or at least add to the protection provided by fiber. It's also possible that people who eat high-fiber foods also have lower intakes of high-fat foods.

To gain the overall benefits of fibers, public health authorities recommend that adults eat at least 25 to 40 grams in food daily (the American Heart Association recommends 25 to 30 grams), ideally, in combination with a low-fat diet. Of this, about 15 grams should be soluble fiber—sufficient to lower your LDL cholesterol level. But to ingest that amount, you'd have to eat much more than most Americans presently consume. Again, nutraceuticals are the logical solution.

Though fiber supplements are not always tasty, you can try them and see if they help lower your cholesterol. Metamucil and Fiber Plan are fiber supplements that contain psyllium. Nutrim is a fat substitute made from the soluble fiber of oats and barley. There are also foods on the market that are psyllium-enriched and that may make it easy for you to take a daily dose of fiber.

CHAPTER THIRTEEN

Heart Healers
on the Horizon

While in his bath, ancient Greek mathematician and scientist Archimedes noticed that the water level rose as he sank. In an instant, he suddenly realized that his weight was displacing an equal amount of water and that this simple observation offered the answer to a complex problem he had been pondering. Historians say he leapt from the bath and ran naked through the streets crying, "Eureka!" (I have found it!).

Personally, I find this hard to believe—but one never knows.

In any case, researchers seldom make medical discoveries like Archimedes—with a single blinding moment of insight. Besides, Archimedes only happened to be right. It was up to other researchers to confirm the truthfulness of his observation. His type of truthful revelation—in an instant—is uncommon in medicine.

It's true that some medical discoveries appear to be clear-cut: They produce a definitive yes or no answer. But research mostly produces a much less definitive "maybe." Over time, as more studies pile up and are evaluated, these collective "maybes" might be transformed into "probably" or "probably not" and ultimately into a "yes" or "no." The process of turning "maybe" into "yes" can take years. The problem is that most of us, particularly those in the media, abhor "maybe." We don't want to wait for researchers to sort out the evidence. Nutraceuticals frequently fall into the "maybe" zone, with a good possibility of going into the "definite" zone.

I urge you to be patient. Even though I'm a staunch supporter of nutraceuticals, I realize that this is a growing field that needs more research.

Each ingredient in the Cardiac Elixir is backed by years of laboratory and clinical research conducted by professionals. That's why I recommend them. Before too long, there is little doubt that we'll discover many other natural substances that also protect our hearts and provide other health benefits. But it's important to wait until we have strong scientific support—and that means persuasive clinical studies—before making claims for nutraceuticals. In my opinion, some of my more exuberant colleagues who support nutraceuticals are way out in front of science and medicine. I understand the temptation to jump the gun. After all, we're in a very exciting era. But in the long run, the nutraceutical cause just isn't well-served by premature claims.

Still, this book wouldn't be complete without looking ahead to some of the other heart nutraceuticals on the horizon. Many nutraceutical enthusiasts will argue that these substances have already earned the right to be included in the Cardiac Elixir. I'm not so sure. Instead, erring perhaps on the side of caution, I put them in the "promising" category. With that in mind, here's a closer look at a few of these definite "maybes."

Garlic

Garlic is more than just a nutraceutical. I've enjoyed its distinctive flavor in many a fine meal, and I consider it an essential component of good cuisine. But can garlic also lower your risk of heart disease?

It's certainly true that people in southern European countries such as Italy and Greece—the so-called Mediterranean Diet countries—traditionally consume more raw and cooked garlic than we do, and they also have lower rates of cardiovascular disease. But that lower rate might be due to any number of factors other than garlic.

Beyond this, a considerable body of clinical evidence suggests that garlic may lower cholesterol, lower blood pressure, and interfere with platelet aggregation, which is good for preventing blood clots of the kind that cause strokes and other health problems. Research also indicates that garlic may have antioxidant properties and benefit your immune system.

The trouble is, there's also some good research that suggests that garlic doesn't do any of these things.

What Garlic May Do for You

Garlic has many active ingredients, so it's difficult to tease out exactly which ones benefit the heart. The prime contender could be alliin, a sulphur-containing compound. When crushed or cut, garlic's alliin turns into another substance called allicin, which gives garlic its characteristic odor. I say "could be" because researchers can't find allicin in your blood after you've eaten garlic, so they can't confirm that this substance has its supposed effects. Apart from allicin, garlic also contains vitamin C and selenium, which also may have heart-protecting qualities.

Garlic may protect your blood vessels by increasing the activity of an enzyme that regulates the production of nitric oxide—a substance that enables arteries to relax. Garlic also contains ajoene, an anti-clotting substance formed when allicin decomposes in your digestive tract.

In addition, garlic may reduce the fat content of arterial cells, preventing lipids from building up in them. Garlic is also a diuretic; by making you excrete excess fluids and salt, it could lower your blood pressure. On top of this, animal and clinical studies have found that garlic can make certain arteries dilate, thereby increasing bloodflow and protecting the cells lining your blood vessels from being damaged by cholesterol. There's even a preliminary report that garlic may lower the serum level of homocysteine—an emerging risk factor for heart disease and stroke.

The studies of garlic come from around the world. It's truly an international nutraceutical. A broad spectrum of studies supports garlic as a cardio-protector. Here's a summary of the leading research.

■ *A comprehensive analysis of 13 of these studies found that people who ate one to three fresh cloves daily reduced their blood cholesterol levels by 10 percent. In addition, they had a 16 percent drop in their "bad" LDL (low-density lipoprotein) cholesterol and nearly a 7 percent drop in their blood pressure.*

■ *Five different studies conducted over the past 10 years suggest that people taking 600 milligrams to 1,000 milligrams of garlic supplements daily—the amount you'd get in one clove a day, depending on the preparation—lowered their total cholesterol levels by an average of 9 percent.*

■ *Another meta-analysis, conducted in England and combining the findings of six different studies, showed a significant falloff in the overall serum cholesterol levels of thousands of people taking garlic supplements.*

■ *A placebo-controlled, double-blind study published in the* American Journal of Clinical Nutrition *in 1996 by Manfred Steiner, M.D., and his colleagues at Memorial Hospital of Rhode Island reported that aged garlic extract lowered overall cholesterol levels by 6 to 7 percent, their harmful LDL cholesterol by 4 percent, and also had a positive effect on blood pressure. Dr. Steiner's 41 subjects started out with moderately high cholesterol levels and were on a low-fat diet approved by the American Heart Association. So the study demonstrated that garlic could have an effect above and beyond diet. What's something of an issue, though, is that the subjects had to take a relatively large quantity of garlic—*

nine capsules, with 800 milligrams of garlic in each—to show this effect. And 70 percent of the participants could tell the difference between garlic and the placebo, making them less objective—and making the study less definitive.

■ *A clinical German study compared 101 healthy garlic-eating elderly adults, ages 50 to 80, with 101 other elderly people who didn't eat garlic regularly. The results indicated that garlic lowered blood pressure. Not surprisingly, these older subjects tended to have stiff blood vessels, and people with high blood pressure tended to have more hardening of the arteries—but these effects were significantly less among the garlic eaters. Cholesterol levels were similar in both groups, though, which weakens the case for garlic on that score.*

The Case against Garlic

For every study that suggests a positive cardiovascular effect, there seems to be another compelling study suggesting that it has no impact on the heart.

■ *In 1998, the* Journal of the American Medical Association *reported on 25 people with moderately high cholesterol who took 10 milligrams of garlic oil (the equivalent of the oil in 4 to 5 grams of fresh garlic cloves) daily for 4 weeks. The effect? None. In fairness to garlic, however, the study might have been too short.*

■ *Similarly, 900 milligrams of garlic powder daily appeared to have no effect on cholesterol levels in an English study of 115 men and women.*

■ *A study led by J. L. Isaacsohn, M.D., at the Christ Hospital Cardiovascular Research Center in Cincinnati, investigated the effect of the equivalent of one clove of fresh garlic daily on 50 moderate-cholesterol outpatients. They took either a placebo or 2.7 grams of Quai garlic, a brand of garlic powder, for 12 weeks. The garlic powder did not lower cholesterol levels significantly.*

So what should we make of all this?

Garlic may have a far-reaching impact on heart disease, but we need more research to be certain. Perhaps different garlic supplements have different potencies. Perhaps the trick with garlic, as with other nutraceuticals, is to find the right combination. A couple of studies suggest that combining garlic with fish oil, which is mentioned later in this chapter, might be more effective than taking either one separately.

■ *One Canadian study, published by A. J. Adler, Ph.D., of the department of human biology at the University of Guelph in Ontario, examined the effects of garlic and fish oil supplementation alone and in combination of a 12-week period. The subjects were 50 men who had moderately high levels of cholesterol.*

The results, published in the American Journal of Clinical Nutrition, *showed that garlic supplementation alone significantly decreased both total cholesterol and "bad" LDL cholesterol levels. Fish oil supplementation alone decreased triglyceride levels, but also increased LDL levels. The subjects who took both, however, enjoyed the best of both worlds. They had lower cholesterol and triglyceride levels, and the combination cancelled out the rise in LDLs.*

■ *Another study supports this combination. Conducted by N. C. Morcos, M.D., Ph.D., of the division of cardiology at the University of California, Irvine, it examined the effects of fish oil and garlic powder on 40 men with moderately high levels of cholesterol. They showed significant decreases in cholesterol, triglycerides, and LDL levels.*

How to Take Garlic

Some experts think that one to three fresh uncooked garlic cloves every day are your best bet. Uncooked is important, since the heat from cooking tends to destroy the enzyme that produces allicin. But other experts believe that garlic extract (Kyolic garlic) or garlic powder (Quai garlic), are just as effective as fresh garlic. Whatever form you choose, I have to be honest and say that there are still no clear-cut answers on how much you should take. There is no doubt that garlic, in whatever form, could prove to be highly effective. It's just too far into the "maybe" zone to get specific about dosages.

Keep in mind that garlic in large doses can have unpleasant side effects, such as bad breath, abdominal pain, heartburn, flatulence, and even rashes. But even at high levels, garlic appears to be safe.

Omega-3 Fatty Acids

In the film version of Ernest Hemingway's *The Old Man and the Sea*, actor Spencer Tracy as the aging Cuban fisherman speaks for many anglers when he says, "Fish, I respect you and I love you."

Sometimes fishing can be disappointing, as it is at the end of the Hemingway story, when the old man helplessly watches sharks devour his hard-earned catch. But a regular diet of fish may turn out to be one of the best ways to get yourself off the hook from heart disease.

Omega-3 fatty acids, a particular kind of polyunsaturated fat found in fatty fish such as salmon, swordfish, and sardines, has been getting a lot of media coverage as a cure-all for heart disease, rheumatoid arthritis, psoriasis, and a host of autoimmune disorders.

The theory that these fats can reduce the risk of coronary heart disease was originally based on low rates of heart disease among native Alaskans, Japanese, and Greenland Inuit. These cultures all consume a lot more fat and cholesterol from the fish in their diets than we do from all sources, but they still have a lower incidence of heart disease.

What Omega-3's May Do for You

A number of studies suggest that large doses of fish oil may reduce blood pressure, reduce inflammation in blood vessels, keep platelets in your blood from sticking together, and even affect immune function.

There also is a good body of clinical research indicating that fish oil may reduce your blood VLDL (very low density lipoprotein) and triglyceride levels. That may be a good thing, particularly for people with diabetes. On the other hand, some studies show that fish oil may impair blood sugar control in people with non-insulin-dependent diabetes, so it may have the potential for being harmful to certain patients.

The evidence that omega-3's reduce your total blood cholesterol is less convincing. In fact, large doses of fish oil supplement might increase bad LDL cholesterol in some people, particularly those who have high blood concentrations of triglycerides.

The Ambiguous Evidence

On the whole, large-scale studies of fish consumption and its impact on heart disease are inconsistent. But a number of studies report that large doses of fish oil may keep platelets in your blood from sticking together, reduce inflammation in blood vessels, and even reduce your blood pressure. And an increasing body of evidence does seem to demonstrate that omega-3's may reduce your risk of fatal arrhythmias—severely irregular heartbeat rhythms.

■ *The Harvard Health Professionals Follow-Up Study reported in 1995 that fish consumption didn't reduce the risk of heart disease among its subjects but might have reduced their risk of dying from it. Another study looking at 1,800 men in the Chicago area over three decades found that those who ate at least 225 grams of fish (about half a pound) every week were 40 percent less likely to die of a first heart attack than those who ate no fish.*

■ *Still another study—the Physicians' Health Study, published in the* Journal of the American Medical Association *in 1998—reported that men who ate fish at least once a week were 52 percent less likely to suffer sudden cardiac death. Their fish consumption was not connected to the risk of having a heart attack— just the risk of dying from one.*

All these people survived, clinical researchers speculate, because fish oils may be able to prevent fatal arrhythmias. Many studies,

Sources of Omega-3's

What are the best sources of omega-3 fatty acids? They can be found in fish and vegetables, seeds, and seed oils—but the omega-3 fatty acids found in fish seem to be better for your heart. Certain vegetable oils, such as flaxseed oil, as well as a number of leafy greens, contain a *short-chain* omega-3 fatty acid. Some believe that this kind is as beneficial as omega-3 fats from fish, but the evidence is not as good. Evidence is on the side of the kind of *longer chain* omega-3 fatty acids found in fish.

Here's a list of some foods—including fish, vegetables, and vegetable products—that contain large amounts of these substances, which many researchers believe are beneficial to the cardiovascular system.

Arugula	Kale
Canola oil	Mackerel
Chicory	Salmon
Chilean sea bass	Sardines
Collard greens	Swiss chard
Endive	Swordfish
Flax bread	Tuna
Flaxseed	Walnut oil
Flaxseed oil	Walnuts
Herring	Watercress

mostly in animals, bear out this hypothesis. It seems that when your red blood cells have a relatively low amount of omega-3 fatty acids, you are at much greater risk of cardiac arrest (from a fatal arrhythmia) than someone whose red blood cell omega-3 fatty acids are at higher levels.

But any number of factors can account for this reduction other than omega-3's. It could be, for instance, that eating less saturated fat—as you are apt to do when you substitute fish for red meat—may be healthier for the heart than any special effects of fish oil.

I'd like to see more clinical evidence supporting fish oil before I agree not to object to its use as a supplement. In the meantime, as a dietary addition, I believe that eating fish is certainly a good idea. A couple of servings of fish every week is an important component of any healthy diet. It contains less fat than many other forms of high-protein foods, it may reduce your triglyceride level, and it may even have an effect similar to aspirin in reducing your risk of heart attack.

How to Take Fish Oil

Obviously, fish itself can be bought in grocery stores or fish markets. The fresher, the better: The omega-3 fatty acids in fish deteriorate quickly in the presence of oxygen and light. Fish oil capsules are available in pharmacies and health food stores. Adults might consider 2 to 3 grams daily of fish oil, or up to three fish meals weekly.

Keep in mind, however, that in large doses, fish oil can cause diarrhea, nausea, and bad breath. Like garlic, fish oil can also decrease blood clotting, which means that people who have clotting problems or who are taking blood-thinning medications should steer clear of fish oil supplements.

Vitamin C

Linus Pauling, one of the twentieth century's great scientific mavericks, professed an almost fanatical devotion to vitamin C in the last 25 years of his life. According to Pauling, vitamin C could cure the common cold, cancer, and a host of other serious ailments. In fact, Pauling suggested that vitamin C could prevent atherosclerosis and heart disease by inhibiting the accumulation of plaque on artery walls.

It's hard to argue with a two-time Nobel prize winner. But to a certain extent, I must.

To date, the evidence of vitamin C's ability to reduce cardiovascular disease is disappointing.

What Vitamin C May Do for You

Vitamin C is a water-soluble vitamin found in many foods, including citrus fruits, pineapple, tomatoes, broccoli, peppers, potatoes, Brussels sprouts, and leafy greens. It is crucial for manufacturing collagen, the main protein substance in your body, which forms the framework of blood vessels. Vitamin C, also called ascorbic acid, is also important for keeping your immunity up.

Some researchers think that vitamin C can keep your artery walls more relaxed. And its role as your body's collagen manufacturer could mean that it can strengthen the flexibility of your arteries.

Certainly, vitamin C is good for you. Remember scurvy? But it's cardio-protective effects are still in dispute.

The Case for Vitamin C

A number of researchers report that people deficient in vitamin C are more likely to develop plaque in their arteries and that the higher the vitamin C content in your blood, the lower your cholesterol levels and the higher your good HDL (high-density lipoprotein) levels.

■ *One 12-year study found that people low in vitamin C were twice as likely to develop coronary heart disease.*

■ *Two other studies of healthy people reported that those who were deficient in vitamin C were also more at risk of eventually developing elevated blood pressure, coronary heart disease, and even cerebrovascular strokes.*

■ *Other studies have looked at the effects of vitamin C on arteries. One, conducted at Brigham and Women's Hospital's vascular medicine and atherosclerosis unit in Boston, measured the bloodflow of 12 people with high cholesterol and 12 with normal levels of cholesterol before and after injecting vitamin C into their arteries. The vitamin C improved the bloodflow and widened the blood vessels of people with high cholesterol but didn't affect those with normal cholesterol levels. Only further studies will show whether this effect is beneficial.*

■ *Another study, led by Gary Plotnick, M.D., who specializes in cardiovascular diseases at Baltimore's University of Maryland Medical Center, measured bloodflow after people ate a high-fat meal with and without vitamins C and E. Four hours after the meal, the arteries of people without vitamins had widened by 8 percent. Those who took the vitamins: 18 percent.*

■ *There's also a body of work looking at the effect of vitamin C on the arteries of people with heart failure, which tend to be more constricted than those of healthy people. Theoretically, vitamin C should be good for these people. A German research team led by Burkhard Hornig, M.D., of the cardiology department at the Medizinische Hochschule Hannover, tested this out. They gave 15 patients who had chronic heart failure as well as 8 healthy volunteers vitamin C either by injection or orally for 4 weeks, then measured their artery diameter and bloodflow. The blood vessels of the people with heart failure who had taken vitamin C were measurably more dilated; vitamin C didn't seem to have this effect on healthy people.*

The Case against Vitamin C

Not all the research on heart disease prevention is positive.

■ *The Nurses' Health Study, which has been looking at the health of more than 80,000 women since 1980, found no effect of vitamin C on heart disease rates after adjusting for vitamin E intake.*

■ *Double-blind clinical studies examining whether high doses of vitamin C can lower blood cholesterol have been inconsistent.*

■ *At least one major review of the role of antioxidant vitamins in the prevention of cardiovascular diseases found that the data on vitamin C were inconclusive.*

And even though Dr. Pauling was a proponent of high doses— he once told an interviewer that he took up to 300 times the Recommended Dietary Allowance of the vitamin each day—European studies suggest that excess vitamin C might actually promote free radical damage in the arteries and heart.

How to Take Vitamin C

Although vitamin C's ability to prevent heart disease is uncertain, everyone, healthy or sick, should take the RDA of 60 milligrams daily, preferably in food, for overall health. In large doses, vitamin C could have negative effects, possibly including excessive absorption of iron for some people, gastrointestinal upset, and increased risk of kidney stones.

Beta-Carotene

Not long ago, beta-carotene was hot news. Studies suggested that it prevented oral cancer, delayed the formation of cataracts, and reduced the risk of heart attack. But that was then; this is now.

The early excitement about beta-carotene has ebbed. Further research has found that beta-carotene may not protect the heart as much as once believed.

What Beta-Carotene May Do for You

Beta-carotene is a member of the carotenoid family of nutrients that is converted into vitamin A in your body. Vitamin A has many functions, including maintaining good vision and bone growth. It's easy to recognize the foods that contain carotenes. They are nature's pigments, and they come in shades of red, orange, and yellow. Carotene is also in most green leaves, becoming visible only in the fall, when the green fades and other colors appear. Beta-carotenes are found in apricots, carrots, sweet potatoes, squash, watermelon, guava, tomatoes, green plants, and green peppers.

An antioxidant, beta-carotene may protect against disease by neutralizing unstable oxygen molecules, called free radicals, in your body.

The Case for Beta-Carotene

Beta-carotene has proven effective in some studies.

■ *The Health Professionals Follow-Up Study, which provided such convincing evidence for the effectiveness of vitamin E, also suggested an association between high beta-carotene intake and less risk of heart disease. But the association only held among current and former smokers. Beta-carotene didn't seem to protect the hearts of nonsmokers.*

■ *Another study of 1,299 nursing home residents in the United States did suggest a heart-health benefit from a high dietary intake of beta-carotene.*

■ *A number of other studies have found that people who have higher levels of beta-carotene are less at risk of getting heart disease.*

The Case against Beta-Carotene

Now, for the cons.

The Nurses' Health Study found no heart-protective effects for beta-carotene once intake for vitamins E and C was considered. Neither did a large study of postmenopausal women in the United States, and neither did the Physicians' Health Study.

Furthermore, the same major review of antioxidant vitamins that dismissed vitamin C for the prevention of cardiovascular diseases also reports that large, randomized clinical trials of beta-carotene show no effect and may even demonstrate a potential for harm.

■ *One major trial found that total mortality was 8 percent higher among people who were taking 20 milligrams of beta-carotene daily.*

■ *Another trial on more than 18,000 smokers called the Beta-Carotene and Retinol Efficacy Trial was called to a halt early because the people taking beta-carotene and vitamin A started showing a statistically significant increase in lung cancer. In my opinion, this may or may not be true.*

What's happening? One new theory is that high doses of beta-carotene are harmful because they interfere with some of the beneficial activities of vitamin C.

How to Take Beta-Carotene

At this point, the scientific evidence to support beta-carotenes as a cardiovascular nutraceutical is not strong. However, they are important for your health in general. For example, they are essential to keep your immune system at its best. In any case, the foods that are rich in beta-carotenes—primarily red, yellow, and orange vegetables—are all healthful. So make them a central part of your diet.

As I don't recommend beta-carotene as a preventative for cardiovascular disease, I therefore have no position on much you need to take.

Coenzyme Q_{10}

Coenzyme Q_{10} certainly looks good in studies conducted in scientific laboratories. It belongs to a class of substances called ubiquinones, which are in every cell of your body and in every cell of every species of plant or animal on the planet. In fact, the prefix "ubi" is short for "ubiquitous."

Unfortunately, there's so much hype about coenzyme Q_{10}, also known as CoQ_{10}, that it's hard for consumers to know what to believe. Keep in mind, thought, that 12 million people in Japan now take coenzyme Q_{10} every day, convinced that it will protect them against many forms of heart disease. And Japanese physicians agree.

So what's the truth? I'll try to sort it out for you.

What Coenzyme Q_{10} May Do for You

Like carnitine, coenzyme Q_{10} helps your heart cells create energy. And like carnitine, it's an essential component of your cells' mitochondria—the "furnaces" in each cell.

In your body, coenzyme Q_{10} attaches itself easily to cell membranes. From there, it moves into your cells' mitochondria. There, it aids in cell respiration and acts as a vital catalyst in the formation of adenosine triphosphate (ATP)—the truly miraculous molecule that produces energy for your cells.

Because all cellular function depends on having enough ATP, you would die without your coenzyme Q_{10}. Low levels of this substance in your body, therefore, are bad for you and may be especially bad for your heart. Low levels of coenzyme Q_{10} have been reported to be associated with many coronary ailments, including angina, high blood pressure, and congestive heart failure.

In addition, coenzyme Q_{10} may keep your LDL cholesterol levels down and alleviate symptoms of cardiomyopathy and angina.

The Ambiguous Evidence

At the Ninth International Conference on coenzyme Q_{10} in Italy in 1996, scientists around the world were reporting on a growing body of clinical evidence supporting the contention that this substance is essential for fueling and therefore strengthening the heart and other muscles. Proponents also believe that coenzyme Q_{10} has powerful antioxidant properties, especially in conjunction with vitamin E.

The trouble is that so far, very little of this good clinical evidence has been published in first-class journals. And much of the research has been conducted on relatively small groups of people. There's enough out there to tantalize the skeptics, but not enough to completely convince me that coenzyme Q_{10} is an effective preventative for heart disease.

Here's what we know.

Cardiomyopathy and Congestive Heart Failure

Cardiomyopathy is a catch-all term describing the condition wherein your heart is too weak to work efficiently as a pump. It means that your heart cells are not strong enough to adequately pump the blood that is present in the heart chambers.

Given that coenzyme Q_{10} is responsible for helping your heart produce energy through ATP—and that there's a strong and consistent correlation between low blood and tissue levels of a coenzyme Q_{10} and the severity of heart failure—it only makes sense that coenzyme Q_{10} supplementation might be able to help people with congestive heart failure.

■ *In one preliminary study, 17 patients with mild congestive heart failure took 30 milligrams of coenzyme Q_{10} daily. Within 4 weeks, each and every one of them had improved, and 53 percent were completely without symptoms.*

■ *In one large study in Italy, 2,664 patients took 50 to 150 milligrams of coenzyme Q_{10} daily for 90 days. More than half the patients were reported to improve from at least three symptoms of congestive heart failure. Their skin became less purple, they had less fluid retention, and they had less fluid buildup in their lungs.*

■ *In another study of 126 cardiomyopathy patients who took 100 milligrams of coenzyme Q_{10} daily, 71 percent of them were reported to have significantly improved after 3 months, and 16 percent improved in 6 months. By the end of the 5-year study, 87 percent of these people had improved.*

■ *Finally, a team of Danish researchers led by A. M. Soja, M.D., of Copenhagen's County Hospital Department of Medicine, conducted a comprehensive analysis of eight different studies in which coenzyme Q_{10} was given to a total of more than 350 people with congestive heart failure. The analysis found a statistically significant improvement in seven different symptoms of the disease.*

■ *The research is not always consistent, though. In one well-regarded study, for instance, 79 patients who had congestive heart failure were given either 100 milligrams of coenzyme Q_{10} or a placebo for 3 months. The patients taking the coenzyme Q_{10} did slightly improve in their ability to exercise, though the effect was not strong. And they did report some improvement in their quality of life, but again, the difference, though significant, was not large.*

High Blood Pressure

Almost 40 percent of people with high blood pressure are deficient in coenzyme Q_{10}. That's an argument in itself for taking this substance, I suppose. But there have been some studies demonstrating that it appears to lower blood pressure and cholesterol levels within 4 to 12 weeks. Researchers aren't sure exactly how it can have both effects concurrently. Perhaps coenzyme Q_{10}'s ability to lower cholesterol levels and therefore reduce plaque buildup translates into more open blood vessels, which are less prone to high blood pressure.

Heart Protection during Heart Attacks or Heart Surgery

Researchers have also looked into whether coenzyme Q_{10} can alleviate the effects of a heart attack or heart surgery, and the results seem promising. In one study conducted in India, 78 heart attack victims were given coenzyme Q_{10} for 28 days, while another group got a placebo. The coenzyme Q_{10} group reportedly had significantly less incidence of angina and arrhythmias, higher levels of natural antioxidants, and better heart function. And fewer people in the coenzyme Q_{10} group had second heart attacks. These findings, the researchers said, suggest that coenzyme Q_{10} can be protective for people who have had heart attacks if the supplementation is begun within 3 days after the attack.

Another study examined whether coenzyme Q_{10} could help people undergoing coronary artery surgery. Forty patients undergoing elective surgery received either 150 milligrams of coenzyme Q_{10} or a placebo daily for 7 days before their operations. The treatment group was significantly less likely to suffer arrhythmias after surgery.

How to Take Coenzyme Q_{10}

Coenzyme Q_{10} is in many foods, including beef, pork, oily fish such as salmon, spinach, eggs, and wheat germ. Your body can also make it from the raw materials in foods. But supplementation makes sense because:

■ *You can be deficient in coenzyme* Q_{10} *without being obviously sick.*

■ *You make less coenzyme* Q_{10} *in your body as you age.*

■ *Anti-cholesterol statin drugs, such as Mevacor, can lower your body levels of coenzyme* Q_{10}.

The best thing about coenzyme Q_{10} is that it appears to be quite safe. Even at high doses, no negative side effects have been reported. Even though it's still well into the "maybe" zone, the very fact that laboratory studies are good, that so many doctors are prescribing it, and that so many people are using it suggests that it may have exciting potential as a cardiovascular nutraceutical.

Make sure to take coenzyme Q_{10} dissolved in oil or brewer's yeast. The most effective form is a gelatin capsule that contains coenzyme Q_{10} in soybean oil or a chewy wafer combined with fatty acids. The tablets or powdered form of coenzyme Q_{10} are poorly absorbed and likely ineffective. You can buy coenzyme Q_{10} in supermarkets and at health food stores. The doses effective in research studies range from 50 to 300 milligrams daily.

Cardia Salt Alternative

Originally developed in Finland, this product can be used to season your food instead of ordinary table salt. It is comprised of:

■ *Sodium chloride*

■ *Potassium chloride*

■ *Magnesium sulfate*

■ *L-lysine (an amino acid with a sweet taste that masks the bitterness of the potassium and magnesium)*

But before we discuss why I like this product so much, let's review some of the factors that contribute to high blood pressure.

The Minerals That Affect Blood Pressure

More than 600 million people worldwide have hypertension, also known as high blood pressure. Your doctor may even tell you that the older you get, the more likely you'll develop this condition, which increases your risk of heart attack, stroke, and other cardiovascular complications. But despite what you may have heard, high blood pressure isn't necessarily a consequence of aging, nor is it inevitable. Some of the culprits behind the surge of high blood pressure in the over-50 crowd in North America are three important everyday minerals. In addition to magnesium, which is discussed in chapter 10, these minerals are:

Sodium. For many years—well before sufficient clinical data existed—the medical establishment advised the public that limiting salt consumption would lower blood pressure. It seemed logical because sodium (the main mineral in table salt) retains water, and excess water in your system can lead to high blood pressure. The truth, many doctors admit privately, is that the evidence supporting this notion isn't as persuasive as it might appear. A comprehensive analysis of 114 studies, published in the *Journal of the American Medical Association*, came to the conclusion that limiting salt has only a small benefit. In fact, this benefit was significantly less than that of drugs used to treat high blood pressure. Even doctors who are convinced that there is a connection also acknowledge that cutting back on salt in your diet without changing other dietary factors will probably only trigger a modest drop in blood pressure at best—even though this can be important.

Potassium. Interestingly, the typical American diet is just as low in potassium as it is high in sodium. Why? Potassium is found mostly in unprocessed meats, such as fresh chicken, beef, lamb, and pork, as well as fish, fresh fruits, and vegetables. (Bananas and citrus fruits are particularly good sources.) Unfortunately, many Americans don't eat enough of these foods. Instead, most of us eat fast foods and processed foods such as hamburgers and hot dogs, which are loaded with sodium and nearly void of potassium.

Doctors know that potassium is at least as important as sodium for regulating blood pressure. In fact, it's common knowledge among physicians that restricting potassium sometimes makes blood pressure rise, and giving supplements of the mineral to patients with hypertension sometimes helps lower blood pressure. An impressive body of research supports the theory that eating too much sodium combined with ingesting too little potassium is as much a risk factor for cardiovascular disease as diabetes or elevated cholesterol. So to reduce your risk of heart disease, you need to reduce your sodium intake, increase your potassium consumption, or preferably, do both.

How Cardia Salt Alternative May Help You

The trouble is, eating a low-salt diet—like eating a low-fat diet—is easier said than done. The National Institutes of Health and the American Heart Association recommend that you limit your sodium intake to less than 2.4 grams a day, which works out to the equivalent of 1½ teaspoons of table salt daily. Yet most Americans consume about twice that amount. Even if you cut back on sodium, there's no guarantee that you'll be able to lower your blood pressure without potassium and magnesium, two minerals that are difficult to get through diet alone. After all, how many people do you know who would eat five or six bananas every day to keep their potassium levels reasonably high?

This is where Cardia Salt Alternative can help.

The Promising Evidence

Several convincing studies have found that when some people replace ordinary table salt with Cardia Salt Alternative, their blood pressure drops. And while most of the other salt substitutes on the market have a bitter, unpleasant taste, people who have tried Cardia Salt Alternative report that its taste is indistinguishable from regular table salt. Here's a summary of some of the most persuasive studies.

■ *At a FIM Cardiovascular Nutraceuticals conference in November 1997, David H.G. Smith, M.D., director of Orange*

County Heart Institute and Research Center in California as well as the director of research operations in the department of clinical pharmacology and hypertension at the Veterans Affairs Medical Center, discussed a study he had conducted at his facilities in California. In it, 64 patients with mild to moderate hypertension used a salt shaker filled with either Cardia Salt Alternative or regular salt. Both groups were asked to limit their use of "salt" to 6 grams (1½ teaspoons) a day. The people using Cardia Salt Alternative had a reduction of about 4 millimeters in both the systolic (upper) and diastolic (lower) numbers in their blood pressure readings.

■ *At a Council on Geriatric Cardiology meeting in March 1997, Joel Neutel, M.D., assistant professor of medicine at the University of California, Irvine, and director of hypertension and cardiovascular research at the Orange County Heart Institute presented another clinical study involving Cardia Salt Alternative. In his six-week study of 63 hypertensive people, Dr. Neutel substituted Cardia Salt Alternative for table salt. As a result, systolic blood pressure in these individuals dropped by an average of 2.4 millimeters of mercury and diastolic blood pressure dipped 4.7 millimeters.*

■ *Two months later, Paul Welton, M.D., dean of the School of Public Health at Tulane University in New Orleans, presented similar results at the 12th annual Meeting of the American Society for Hypertension. In his 6-week study, conducted at 13 centers nationwide, he found that substitution of Cardia Salt Alternative for regular salt significantly reduced blood pressure in 223 hypertensive individuals.*

Clearly, Cardia Salt Alternative has a promising future. It helps reduce sodium intake while increasing the amount of potassium and magnesium in the diet. The reduction of the sodium/potassium ratio (in other words, less sodium and more potassium), plus the addition of magnesium, is far more effective at lowering blood pressure than reducing sodium intake alone.

Furthermore, Cardia Salt Alternative does not appear to interfere with the effects of any hypertensive medications that people take to control their blood pressure. In fact, using it may be particularly beneficial to people who are taking beta blockers and ACE inhibitors.

But should you use Cardia Salt Alternative if you're healthy and don't have high blood pressure? I think this is a grey zone. In Finland, where it's consumed by a large percentage of the population, reports suggest there is a significant reduction in cardiovascular disease. But whether this is due to Cardia Salt Alternative is unknown. At this time, it seems reasonable for healthy people, particularly those who are obese or have a family history of high blood pressure, to use this substance instead of salt. However, don't go overboard. Cardia Salt Alternative, which is available at most grocery stores and pharmacies, should be used in moderation just like ordinary table salt. Avoid using this product if you have kidney problems.

References

Carnitine

Anand, I. et al. Acute and chronic effects of propionyl-L-carnitine on the hemodynamics, exercise capacity, and hormones in patients with congestive heart failure. *Cardiovasc Drugs Ther* 1998:12. 291–299.

Bartels, G. L. et al. Acute myocardial ischaemia induces cardiac carnitine release in man. *Eur Heart J* 1997; 18: 84–90.

Brevetti, G. et al. Increases in walking distance in patients with peripheral vascular disease treated with L-carnitine: a double-blind, cross-over study. *Circulation* 77, No. 4, 767–773, 1988.

Brevetti, G. et al. Changes in skeletal muscle histology and metabolism in patients undergoing exercise reconditioning: effect of proprionyl-L-carnitine. *Muscle Nerve* 20: 1115–1120, 1997.

Canale et al. Bicycle ergometer and echocardiographic study in healthy subjects and patients with angina pectoris after administration of L-carnitine: semiautomatic computerized analysis of M-mode tracings. *Int J Clin Pharmacol Ther Toxicol.* 1988;26: 221–4.

Cherchi, A. et al. Effects of L-carnitine of exercise tolerance in chronic stable angina: a multicenter, double-blind, randomized, placebo-controlled crossover study. *Int J Clin Pharmacol Ther Toxicol.* 1985;23: 569–72.

Costa, *Andrologia*, 1994.

Deckert, J. Can treatment with propionyl-L-carnitine improve the quality of life in patients with intermittent claudication? *Journal of Family Practice*, June 1997. Vol. 44, No. 6, p533(2).

DeSimone, C. et al. High dose L-carnitine improves immunologic and metabolic parameters in AIDS patients. *Immunopharmacology and Immunotoxicology*, 1993; 15: 1–2.

DeSimone, C. et al. L-carnitine deficiency in AIDS patients. *AIDS* 1992; 7 (2)j; 203–205

DiPalma, J. L-carnitine: Its therapeutic potential. *American Family Physician.* Dec. 1986. 34(6) 127–30.

Ferrari, R. et al. The effect of L-carnitine on myocardial metabolism of patients with coronary artery disease. *Clin Trials J.* 1984;21: 40–58.

Ferrari, R. et al. The metabolical effects of L-carnitine in angina pectoria. *Int J Cardiol* 1984;5: 213–216.

Iliceto et al. Effects of L-carnitine administration on left ventricular remodeling after acute anterior myocardial infarction: the L-Carnitine Ecocardiografia Digitalizzata Infarto Miocardio (CEDIM) trial. *American College of Clinical Cardiology* 1995; 26: 380–7.

Ioannis Rizos, submitted for publication

Jacoba, K. et al. Effect of L-carnitine on the limitation of infarct size in one-month postmyocardial infarction cases: A multicenter, randomised, parallel, placebo-controlled trial. *Clinical Drug Investigation*, 11 (2) 1996. P. 90–96

Kawikawa, T. et al. Effect of L-carnitine of exercise tolerance in patients with stable angina pectoris. *Jpn Heart J.* 1984;25: 587–597.

Kendler, B. S. Carnitine: An overview of its role in preventative medicine. *Preventative Medicine* 15, 373–390 (1986).

Kosolcharoen, P. et al. Improved exercise tolerance after administration of carnitine. *Curr Ther Res.* 1981;30:753–64.

Menchini et al, *Fertil Steril*, 1984.

Miehe, K. et al. *Carnitine Pathochemical Basics and Clinical Applications.*

Paulson, D. J. Carnitine deficiency-induced cardiomyopathy. *Mol Cell Biochem* 1998 Mar.;180(1–2): 33–41.

Pepine, C. J., The therapeutic potential of carnitine in cardiovascular disorders. *Clinical Therapeutics*, Vol. 13, No. 1, Excerpta Medica, 1991. P. 1–21.

Pons, R. et al. Deficient muscle carnitine transport in primary carnitine deficiency. *Pediatr Res.* 42: 583–587, 1997.

Reforzo, G. et al. Effects of high doses of L-carnitine on myocardial lactate balance during pacing-induced ischemia in aging subject. *Curr Ther Res.* 1986; 40: 374–83.

Sachan, D.S. et al. *Vegetarian Nutrition: An International Journal* (1997) 64–69.

Shug, A. L. et al. Changes in tissue levels of carnitine and other metabolites during myocardial ischemia and anoxia. *Arch Biochem Biophys.* 1978;187: 25–33.

Singh, R.B. et al. A randomized, double-blind, placebo-controlled trial of L-carnitine in suspected acute myocardial infarction. *Postgraduate Medical Journal*, 1996: 72: 45–50.

Thomsen, J. H. et al. Improved pacing tolerance of the ischemic human myocardium after administration of carnitine. *Am J Cardiol.* 1979;43: 300–306.

Vick et al, Pharmacodynamics and therapeutics, *Life Sci. Adv.* 1990; 9: 1–5.

B Vitamins

Alfthan, G. et al. Plasma homocysteine and cardiovascular disease mortality. *The Lancet.* Vol. 349, p. 397. Feb. 8, 1997.

Arneson, E., Refsum, H., Bonaa, K. H., Ueland, P. M., Forde, O. H., Nordrehaug, J. E. Serum total homocysteine and coronary heart disease. *Int J Epidemiol.* 1995;24: 704–709.

Boushey, C. J., Beresford, S. A., Omen, G. S., Motulsky, A. G. A quantitative assessment of plasma homocysteine as a risk factor for vascular disease. Probable benefits of increasing folic acid intakes. *JAMA* 1995:274: 1049–57.

Brattström, Lars. Vitamins as homocysteine-lowering agents, *J. Nutr.* 126: 1276S–1280S. 1996.

Broihier, K. Change of heart: new research suggests folate, B_6 are keys to a healthy heart. *Food Processing.* May 1998. 59(5). 60.

Brown, E. W. Folate, B_{12}, and B_6 for the heart. *Medical Update.* Mar. 1998. 21(9).1, 2.

Clarke, R. Lowering blood homocysteine with folic acid based supplements: meta-analysis of randomised trials. *JAMA.* June 3, 1998. 279(21) 1678E(1).

Colloquium: Homocyst(e)ine, vitamins, and arterial occlusive diseases. *J. Nutr.* 126: 1273S–1275S. 1996–2000.

Editorial: Folate and cardiovascular disease: why we need a trial now. *JAMA*, June 26, 1996. 275 (24) 1929–30.

Editorial: Homocysteine, folate, vitamin B_6, and cardiovascular disease. *JAMA*, Feb. 4, 1998. 279(5) 392.

Fallest-Strobl, P. C. et al. Homocysteine: a new risk factor for atherosclerosis. *American Family Physician.* Oct. 15, 1997.

Folsom, A. R. et al. Prospective study of coronary heart disease incidence in relation to fasting total homocysteine, related genetic polymorphisms, and B vitamins: the Atherosclerosis Risk in Communities (ARIC) study. *Circulation.* 1998;98: 204–210.

Graham, I. et al. Plasma homocysteine as a risk factor for vascular disease: European Concerted Action Project. *JAMA*, June 11, 1997. 277(22) 1775–1781.

Guttormsen, A. B. et al. Determinants and vitamin responsiveness of intermediate hyperhomocysteinemia: The Hordaland Homocysteine Study. *J. Clin. Invest.* Nov. 1996. 98 (9). 2174–83.

Hofmann et al. Hyperhomocyst(e)inemia and endothelial dysfunction in IDDM. *Diabetes Care*, Vol. 20, No. 13, Dec. 1997. 1880–1886.

Homocysteine Lowering Trialists' Collaboration. Lowering blood homocysteine with folic acid based supplements: meta-analysis of randomised trials. *BMJ.* Mar. 21, 1998. 316. 894–898.

Ma, J. et al. Methylenetetrahydrofolate reductase polymorphism, plasma folate, homocysteine, and risk of myocardial infarction in U.S. physicians. *Circulation.* 1996; 94: 2410–2416.

Malinow, M. R. et al. Reduction of plasma homocyst(e)ine levels by breakfast cereal fortified with folic acid in patients with coronary heart disease. *N Engl J Med.* 1998; 338: 1009–15.

Mason, Joel B. and Joshua W. Miller, The effects of vitamin B_{12}, B_6, and folate on blood homocysteine levels.

McCully, K. S. Relationship of dietary folate and vitamin B_6 with coronary heart disease in women (letter to the editor). *JAMA*. Aug. 5, 1998. 280 (5). 419.

Morrison, H., et al. Serum folate and risk of fatal coronary heart disease. *JAMA*, June 26, 1996. Vol. 275, No. 24. 1893–1896.

Nygård, O. et al. Plasma homocysteine levels and mortality in patients with coronary artery disease. *N Engl J Med*. 1997;337: 230–6.

Petri, M., et al. Plasma homocysteine as a risk factor for atherothrombotic events in systemic lupus erythematosis. *The Lancet*. Vol. 348. Oct. 26, 1996.

Rimm, E. et al. Folate and vitamin B_6 from diet and supplements in relation to risk of coronary heart disease among women. *JAMA*, Feb. 4, 1998, Vol. 279, No. 5: 359–364.

Robinson, K. et al. Low circulating folate and vitamin B_6 concentrations: risk factors for stroke, peripheral vascular disease, and coronary artery disease. *Circulation*. 1998;97: 437–43.

Selheeb et al, *N. Eng. J. Med.*, 1995–lupus erythenatosus and stroke study, showing that increased homocysteine levels are associated with increased stroke and thrombis formation.

Selhub, J. et al, Plasma homocysteine and extrasetanial carotid stenosis in the Framingham Heart Study. *N. Eng. J. Med.*, 1995. 332: 286–291.

Soo-Sang Kang. Treatment of hyperhomocyst(e)inemia: physiological basis. *J. Nutri*. 126: 1273S–1275S. 1996.

Stampfer, M. et al. A prospective study of plasma homocysteine and risk of myocardial infarction in U.S. physicians. *JAMA*, Aug. 19, 1992. Vol. 268, No. 7: 877–881.

Stein, J. H. Hyperhomocysteinemia and atherosclerotic vascular disease. *Arch Intern Med*. 1998;158: 1301–1306.

Wald, N. et al. Homocysteine and ischemic heart disease: results of a prospective study with implications regarding prevention. *Arch Intern Med*. 1998;158 (8). 862–867.

Vitamin E

Azen et al. Effect of supplementary antioxidant vitamin intake on carotid arterial wall intima-media thickness in a controlled clinical trial of cholesterol lowering. *Circulation* 1996; 94: 2369–2372.

Beach et al. 1992 Specific nutrient abnormalities in asymptomatic HIV-1 infection. *AIDS* 6: 701–8.

Bellizzi, M. C. et al. Vitamin E and coronary heart disease: The European Paradox. *Eur J Clin Nutr* 48, 822–831, 1994.

Blot et al. Nutrition intervention trials in Linxian, China: supplementation with specific vitamin/mineral combinations, cancer incidence, and disease-specific mortality in the general population. *J. Natl Cancer Inst*. 1993. 85: 1483–92.

Chirico, G. et al. 1983. Deficiency of neutrophil phagocytosis in premature infants: effect of vitamin E supplementation. *Acta Paeditr Scand* 72: 521–4.

Diplock, A. T. Antioxidant nutrients and disease prevention: an overview. *Am J. Clin Nutr*. Jan. 1991;53: 189S–93S.

Gey, K. F., Moser, U. K. et al. Increased risk of cardiovascular disease at suboptimal plasma concentrations of essential antioxidants: an epidemiological update with special attention to carotene and vitamin C. *Am.J.Clin.Nutr*. 1993: 57(suppl): 787S–97S.

Gey, K. F. et al. Inverse correlation between plasma vitamin E and mortality from ischemic heart disease in cross-cultural epidemiology. *Am J Clin Nutr*. 53, 326S–334S, 1991.

Gey, K. F. Plasma levels of antioxidant vitamins in relation to ischemic heart disease and cancer. *Am J Clin Nutri*. May #5 Suppl. 1987;43: 1368–77.

Heinonen, O. P. and Huttunen, J. K. et al. The Alpha-Tocopherol, Beta-Carotene Cancer Prevention Study Group. The effect of vitamin E and beta carotene on the incidence of lung cancer and other cancers in male smokers. *N Engl J Med* 1994: 330: 1029–35.

Hodis, H. N., Mack, W. J., LaBree, L., Cashin-Hemphil, L., Sevanian, A. et al. Serial coronary angiographic evidence that antioxidant vitamin intake reduces progression of coronary artery atherosclerosis. *J. Am. Med Assoc*. 1995; 273: 1849–1854.

Hodis, H. N. et al. Serial angiographic evidence that antioxidant vitamin intake reduces progression of coronary artery atherosclerosis. *JAMA*. 1995; 273: 1849–54.

Knekt, P. et al. Antioxidant vitamin intake and coronary mortal-ity in a longitudinal population study. *Am J Epidemiol*. 1994: 139: 1180–9.

Kushi et al. Intake of vitamins A, C, and E and postmenopausal breast cancer. The Iowa Women's Health Study. *Am J Epidemiol.* 1996. 144: 165–74.

Manson, J. E. et al. A prospective study of antioxidant vitamins and incidence of coronary heart disease in women. *Supplement II Circulation.* Oct. 1991. 84(4). 2169.

Meydani, S. N. et al. Assessment of the safety of supplementation with different amounts of vitamin E in healthy older adults. *Am J Clin Nutr* 1998; 68: 311–8.

Meydani, S. N. et al. Recent developments in vitamin E and immune response. *Nutrition Reviews.* Vol. 56 (1). S49–S58.

Passi et al. Study on plasma polyunsaturated phospholipids and vitamin E, and on erythrocyte glutathione peroxidase in high risk HIV infection categories and AIDS patients. *Clin Chem Enzymol Commun* 5. 1993: 169–77.

Rimm, E. B. et al. Vitamin E consumption and the risk of coronary heart disease in men. *N. Eng. J. Med.* May 29, 1993. 328(20) 1450–6.

Stampfer, M. J. and Rimm, E. B. Epidemiologic evidence for vitamin E in prevention of cardiovascular disease. *Am J Clin Nutr.* 1995;62(suppl): 1365S–9S.

Steiner, M. et al., Vitamin E plus aspirin compared with aspirin alone in patients with transient ischemic attacks. *American Journal of Clinical Nutrition.* 62 (6 Suppl), Dec. 1995: 1381S–1384S.

Stephens, N. G. et al. Randomised controlled trial of vitamin E in patients with coronary disease: Cambridge Heart Antioxidant Study (CHAOS). *The Lancet.* 1996; 347: 781–86.

Tavier et al. 1994. Antioxidant status and lipid peroxidatin in patients infected with HIV. *Chem Biol Interact* 91: 165–80.

Taylor et al. 1994. Prevention of esophageal cancer: the nutrition intervention trials in Llinxian, China. Linxian Nutrition Intervention Trials Study Group. Cancer Re 54 (suppl): 2029S–31.

Verhoeven et al. 1997. Vitamins C and E, retinol, beta-carotene, and dietary fibre in relation to breast cancer risk: a prospective cohort study. *Brit J Cancer.* 75: 149–55.

Alcohol

AHA press release, Feb. 7, 1997.

Camargo, C. A. Jr., Stampfer, M. J., Glynn, R. J. et al. Moderate alcohol consumption and risk for angina pectoris or myocardial infarction in U.S. male physicians. *Arch Intern Med* 126(5): 372–5, 1997 Mar. 1.

Camargo, C. A. Jr, Stampfer, M. J., Glynn, R. J. et al. Prospective study of moderate alcohol consumption and risk of peripheral arterial disease in U.S. male physicians. *Circulation* 95(3): 577–80, 1997 Feb. 4.

Cestaro et al, 1996.

Chenet, L. et al. Alcohol and cardiovascular mortality in Moscow, new evidence of a causal association. *J. Epidemiol. Comm. Health.* 1998; 52: 772–74.

Chou et al. Medical consequences of alcohol consumption—United States, 1992. *Alcohol Clin Exp Res.* Vol 20, No. 8, 1996: 1423–1429.

Criqui et al. The French paradox: Does diet or alcohol explain the difference? *The Lancet.* 2, 1994.

Dorozynski, Al. Moderate wine drinking reduces all cause mortality. *BMJ.* 316. Feb. 28 1998.

Gaziano, J. M., Buring, J. E., Breslow, J. L. et al. Moderate alcohol intake, increased levels of high-density lipoprotein and its subfractions, and decreased risk of myocardial infarction. *N Engl J Med* 329(25): 1829–34, 1993 Dec. 16.

Jackson, R et al. Does recent alcohol consumption reduce the risk of acute myocardial infarction and coronary death in regular drinkers? *Am J Epidemiol.* 136: 819, 1992.

Kannel, William B, Ellison, R. Curtis. Alcohol and coronary heart disease: the evidence for a protective effect. *Clinica Chimica Acta* 246 (1996) 59–76.

Lazarus, R., Sparrow, D., Weiss, S. T. Alcohol intake and insulin levels in men: Evidence for lower insulin resistance in moderate drinkers from the Normative Aging Study. *Am J Epidemiol* 1997;145(10): 909–916.

Maclure, M. Demonstration of deductive meta-analysis: ethanol intake and risk of myocardial infarction. *Epidemiologic Reviews.* 1993. 15(2) 328–51.

McKee, M. and Leon, D. Letter to the editor: Global epidemic of cardiovascular disease. *The Lancet.* Feb. 6, 1999. (353). 503.

Mihic, S. J. et al. Sites of alcohol and volatile anaesthetic action on GABA(A) and glycine receptors. *Nature.* 1997 Sep 25; 389(6649): 385–9.

Moore, R. D., Pearson, T. A. Moderate alcohol consumption and coronary artery disease. *Medicine.* 1986; 65: 242–67.

Muntwyler, J. et al, Mortality and light to moderate alcohol consumption after myocardial infarction. *The Lancet.* Vol 352, Dec. 12, 1998: 1882–1885.

Pearson, T. A. et al. *JAMA.* 1994; 272: 967–68.

Ridker, P. M. et al. *JAMA.* 1994; 272: 929–33.

Rimm, E. et al. Folate and vitamin B_6 from diet and supplements in relation to risk of coronary heart disease among women. *JAMA*, Feb. 4, 1998, Vol. 279, No. 5: 359–364.

Rimm, E. et al. Prospective study of alcohol consumption and risk of coronary disease in men. *The Lancet.* 1991. Aug. 24; 338 (8765) 464–8.

Rimm, E. et al. Review of moderate alcohol consumption and reduced risk of coronary heart disease: is the effect due to beer, wine, or spirits? *BMJ.* Mar. 1996. 312 (7033). 731–6.

Sacco, R. L. The protective effect of moderate alcohol consumption on ischemic stroke. *JAMA.* 1999; 281: 53–60.

Smith-Warner, S. A. et al. Alcohol and breast cancer in women: a pooled analysis of cohort studies. *JAMA.* Feb. 18, 1998. 279. 535–540.

Stampfer, M. J. et al. A prospective study of moderate alcohol consumption and the risk of coronary disease and stroke in women. *N. Engl J. Med.* 1988; 319: 267–73.

Thorton, J. et al. Moderate alcohol intake reduces bile cholesterol saturation and raises HDL cholesterol. *The Lancet*, 1983: 819–22.

Thun, Michael J. et al. Alcohol consumption and mortality among middle-aged and elderly U.S. adults. *N. Engl J. Med.*, Vol. 337, Number 24: 1705–1714.

Truelsen et al. *Stroke: Journal of the American Heart Association.* Dec. 1998 issue. Copenhagen City Heart Study.

Yu, H. Letter to the editor: Alcohol consumption and breast cancer risk. *JAMA.* Oct.7, 1998; 280: 1138–1139.

Zhang, Y. et al. Light drinking does not appear to be a risk factor for breast cancer. *American Journal of Epidemiology.* Jan. 15, 1999; 149: 93–105.

Magnesium

Abraham, A. et al. *N. Engl J. Med.* 296: 862–63, 1977.

Alltur, B. T. et al. Magnesium dietary intake modulates blood lipid levels and atherogenesis. *Proc Nat Acad Sci USA.* 1990: 87: 1840–44.

Altura, B. M. et al. Magnesium and the cardiovascular system: experimental and clinical aspects updated. In: Sigel H, Sigel A., Eds. Compendium on Magnesium and its role in biology, nutrition, and physiology. *Met. Ions Biol Syst.* 1990: 26: 359–416.

Altura, B. M. et al. Cardiovascular risk factors and magnesium: relationships to atherosclerosis, ischemic heart disease, and hypertension. *Magnes. Trace Elem.* 1991–92: 10: 182–192.

American Diabetes Association. Magnesium supplementation in the treatment of diabetes. *Diabetes Care.* 1992; 15(8). 1065–1067.

Bashir, Y. et al. Effects of long-term oral magnesium chloride replacement in congestive heart failure secondary to coronary artery disease. *Am J Cardiol.* 1993; 72: 1156–62.

Campbell, R. K., Nadler, J., editors. *Implications of magnesium deficiency in diabetes.* City of Hope Department of Diabetes, Endocrinology and Metabolism. Oct. 1993. Published by BIMARK Inc., New Jersey.

Casscells, W. Magnesium and myocardial infarction. *The Lancet.* 1994; 343: 807–809.

Comstock, G. W. Water hardness and cardiovascular diseases. *Am J Epidemiol.* 1979. 110: 375–400.

Continuing Survey of Food Intake by Individuals 1989 and 1990. U.S. Dept of Agriculture Public Use Data Tape: 1989.

Davi, G. Thromboxane biosynthesis and platelet function in Type II diabetes mellitus. *N. Engl. J. Med.* 1990: 322: 1769–1774.

DiPalma, J. Magnesium replacement therapy. *American Family Practitioner.* July 1990. 2(4) 173–176.

Durlach, J. et al. Magnesium and aging. *Magnesium Research* (1993) 6, 4, 379–394.

Durlach, J. et al. Magnesium and therapeutics. *Magnesium Research.* (1994) 7, 3/4, 313–328.

Durlach, J. New trends in international magnesium research. *Magnesium Research.* 1992 Mar. 5(1)1–4.

Durlach, J. Present and future of magnesium research. *Journal of Japanese Society for Magnesium Research.* 1993, 12, 2: 113–135.

Editorial: Magnesium for myocardial infarction? *The Lancet.* 1991. Sep 14; 338 (8768): 667–8.

Gottlieb, S. S. Importance of magnesium in congestive heart failure. *Am J Cardio.* 1989 Apr. 18; 63(14): 39G–42G.

Gottlieb, S. S. et al. Prognostic importance of the serum magnesium concentration in patients with congestive heart failure. *J. Am Coll Cardiol.* Oct. 1990; 16(4): 827–31.

Gottlieb, S. S. et al. *Am Heart J.* 1993; 125: 1645–1650.

Hwang, D. et al. Insulin increases intracellular magnesium transport in human platelets. *J Clin Endocrinol Metab* 76: 549–553, 1993.

Jeejeebhoy, K. N. et al. Chromium deficiency, glucose intolerance, and neuropathy reversed by chromium supplementation in a patient receiving long-term total parenteral nutrition. *Am J. Clin Nutr.* 30: 531–538, 1977.

Joffres, M. R. et al. Relationship of magnesium intake and other dietary factors to blood pressure: the Honolulu heart study. *Am J Clin Nutr.* 1987 Feb.; 45(2): 469–75.

Kawano, Y. et al. Effects of magnesium supplementation in hypertensive patients. *Hypertension.* 1998;32: 260–265.

Ma, J. et al. Associations of serum and dietary magnesium with cardiovascular disease, hypertension, diabetes, insulin, and carotid arterial wall thickness: the Atherosclerosis Risk in Communities Study. *J. Clin Epidemiol.* 1995. Jul; 48(7) 927–40.

Maclean, R. M. Magnesium and its therapeutic uses: a review. *Am J Med.* 1994; 96: 63–76.

Malayan, S. et al. Magnesium reduces vascular reactivity, thromboxane release and platelet aggregation in non-insulin-dependent diabetics.

Male Health Professionals study. *Diabetes Care* 20 (4): 545, 1997.

Mather, H. M. et al. Hypomagnesaemia in diabetes. *Clinica Chimica Acta.* 1979. 95: 235–242.

Millane, T. A. et al. *Br Med J.* 1992; 68: 441–442.

Mooradian, A. D. Technical review: selected vitamins and minerals in diabetes. *Diabetes Care.* 1994. 17(5). 464–79.

Nadler et al. Intracellular free magnesium deficiency plans a key role in increased platelet reactivity in Type II diabetes mellitus. *Diabetes Care.* Vol. 15, No. 7, July 1992.

Nurses' Health Study. *JAMA.* 277: 472, 1997.

Nutrition Action Newsletter, Dec. 1998

Paolisso, G. et al. Intracellular magnesium and insulin resistance: results in Pima Indians and Caucasians. *J Clin Endocrinol Metab.* 80: 1382–1385, 1995.

Paolisso, G. et al. Changes in glucose turnover parameters and improvement of glucose oxidation after 4-week magnesium administration in elderly non-insulin-dependent (Type II) diabetic patients. *J Clin Endocrinol Metab* 78: 1510–14, 1994.

Rasmuissen, H. S., McNair, P., Norregard, P., Backer, V., Lindeneg, O., Balslev, S., Intravenous magnesium in acute myocardial infarction. *The Lancet* 1986. I: 234–36.

Resnick, L. et al. Cellular ions in hypertension, diabetes, and obesity: a nuclear magnetic resonance spectroscopic study. *Hypertension.* 1991; 17: 951–957.

Resnick, L. et al. Intracellular and extracellular magnesium depletion in Type 2 (non-insulin-dependent) diabetes mellitus. *Diabetologia.* 1993. 36: in press.

Smith, L. F. et al. Intravenous infusion of magnesium sulphate after acute myocardial infarction: effects on arrhythmias and mortality. *Int J Cardiol.* 1986; 12: 175–80.

Teo, K. K. et al. Effects of intravenous magnesium in suspected acute myocardial infarction: overview of randomized trials. *BMJ* 1991. 303 (6816): 1499–503.

Touyz, R. M. Magnesium supplementation as an adjuvant to synthetic calcium channel antagonists in the treatment of hypertension. *Med Hypotheses.* Oct. 1991; 36(2): 140–1.

Woods, K. et al. Long-term outcome after intravenous magnesium sulphate in suspected acute myocardial infarction: the second Leicester Intravenous Magnesium Intervention Trial (LIMIT-2). *The Lancet* 1994; 343: 816–819.

Woods, K. et al. Intravenous magnesium sulphate in suspected acute myocardial infarction: results of the second Leicester Intravenous Magnesium Intervention Trial (LIMIT-2). *The Lancet* 1992; 339: 1553–1558.

Chromium

Anderson, R. et al. Elevated intakes of supplemental chromium improve glucose and insulin variables in individuals with Type 2 diabetes. *Diabetes,* Vol. 46, Nov. 1997: 1786–1791.

Anderson, R. A. Chromium, glucose intolerance, and diabetes. *Journal of the American College of Nutrition.* 1998. 17(6). 548–55.

Anderson, R. A. et al. Supplemental chromium effects on glucose, insulin, glucagon, and urinary chromium losses in subjects consuming controlled low-chromium diets. *Am J Clin Nutr.* 54: 909–916. 1991.

Cefalu, W. T, et al. The effect of chromium supplementation on carbohydrate metabolism and body fat distribution. *Diabetes*. 46 (Suppl.1): 55A, 1997.

Fox, G. N. et al. Chromium picolinate supplementation for diabetes mellitus. *The Journal of Family Practice* 1998. 46(1) 83–86.

Mertz, W. Interaction of chromium with insulin: a progress report. *Nutrition Reviews*. 1999. 56(6) 174–7.

Ravina, A. et al. Clinical use of the trace element chromium (III) in the treatment of diabetes mellitus. *J. Trace Elem. Exp. Med.* 1995; 8: 183–190.

Ravina, A. et al. *Diabetic Medicine.*

Cardia Salt

Alderman, M. et al. Study on the association between low urinary sodium and myocardial infarction *Hypertension*. 1995: 25: 1144.

Gelleijnse, J. M. et al. Reduction in blood pressure with a low sodium, high potassium, high magnesium salt in older subjects with mild to moderate hypertension. *BMJ*. 1994; 309: 456–9.

Karppanen, H. and Mervaala, E., 1996. Adherence to and population impact of non-pharmacological and antihypertensive therapy. *J. Human Hypertension*, 10: S57–S59.

Kawasaki, T., and Itoh, K. 1996. The report on "PanSalt": medical and nutritional studies on the mineral salt "PanSalt." Abstract, *Council on Geriatric Cardiology*.

Law et al. Metroanalysis. *British Medical Journal*. 1991.

Mervaala, E. et al. Cardiovascular effects of felodipine are not antagonized by dietary salt. *European Journal of Pharmacology*, 1994. 225: 73–79.

Mervaala, E. et al. Replacement of regular salt by a novel salt alternative improves the cardiovascular effects of the ACE inhibitor enalapril. *Hypertension Research*, 1994; 17: 59–69.

Mervaala, E. et al. Replacement of salt by a novel potassium-and-magnesium-enriched salt alternative improves the cardiovascular effects of ramipril. *British Journal of Pharmacology*, 1994; 112: 640–8.

Neutel, J., 1996. The effects of replacing regular salt with a reduced-sodium salt containing potassium and magnesium may offer a non-pharmacological approach to lowering blood pressure. Abstract, *American Heart Association*.

Neutel, J. and Smith, D. 1997. The effects of replacing regular salt at the table with a new mineral salt containing reduced sodium and added potassium and magnesium may help lower blood pressure without affecting taste. Abstract, *Council on Geriatric Cardiology*.

Omvik, P., and MyKing, O. L., 1995. Unchanged central hemodynamics after six months of moderate sodium restriction with or without potassium supplement in essential hypertension. *Blood Pressure*, 4: 32–41.

Philips, R. A. et al., 1998. Blood pressure reduction with an antihypertensive program of JNC lifestyle modifications and use of a reduced sodium salt containing potassium and magnesium in patients with hypertension. Abstract, *American Society for Hypertension*.

Rosenfield, A. Host of Expert Panel Proceedings, Dec. 5, 1996, on the role of dietary sodium and potassium in the prevention and management of hypertension: a public concern, at Columbia School of Public Health.

Svetkey et al. Effects of dietary patterns on blood pressure: Subgroup analysis of the Dietary Approaches to Stop Hypertension (DASH) randomized clinical trial. *Archives of Internal Medicine* 1999; 159: 285–293.

Whelton, P. et al. 1997. The use of a reduced-sodium salt containing potassium and magnesium as an adjunctive approach to treatment of hypertension with antihypertensive medications. Abstract, *American Society for Hypertension*.

Whelton, P. K. et al. Science News Update. *JAMA*, 1997; 277: 1624; May 28, 1997; Reuters, May 27.

Whelton, P. K., et al. *JAMA* 1997.

Niacin

Canner, P.L., et al. Fifteen-year mortality in Coronary Drug Project patients; long-term benefit with niacin. *Journal of the American College of Cardiology*. 8:6: Dec. 1986. 1245–1255.

The Coronary Drug Project Group. Clofibrate and niacin in coronary heart disease. *JAMA* 231, 360–381, 1975.

DiPalma, J. R. and Thayer, W. S. Use of niacin as a drug. *Annu Rev Nutr*. 11, 169–187, 1991.

Illingworth, D. R. et al., Comparative effects of lovastatin and niacin in primary hypercholesterolemia. *Arch Intern Med*. 154, 1586–1595, 1994.

McKenney, J. M. et al. A comparison of the efficacy and toxic effects of sustained versus immediate-release niacin in hypercholesterolemic patients. *JAMA*. 271, 672–677, 1994.

Vega, G. L. et al. Lipoprotein responses to treatment with lovastatin, gemfibrozil and nicotinic acid in normalipidemic patients with hypoalphalipoproteinemia. *Arch Intern Med*. 154, 73–82, 1994.

Soy

Adlercreutz, H., Maxur, W. Phyto-oestrogens and Western diseases. The Finnish Medical Society DUODECIM, *Ann Med*, 1997; 29: 95–120.

Adolph, W. H., Kiang, P.C. The nutritional value of soy bean products. *China Med J*. 34: 268–275, 1920.

Anderson, J. W. et al. Meta-analysis of the effects of soy protein intake on serum lipids. *New England Journal of Medicine*. 333: 276–282, Aug. 3, 1995.

Anthony, M. S. et al. Effects of soy isoflavones on atherosclerosis: potential mechanisms. *Am J Clin Nutr* 1998; 6 (suppl): 1390S–3S.

Bakhit, R. M. et al. Intake of 25 g of soybean protein with or without soybean fibers alters plasma lipids in men with elevated cholesterol concentrations. *J Nutr*. 1994; 124: 213–222.

Baum, J. A. et al. Long-term intake of soy protein improves blood lipid profiles and increases mononuclear cell low-density lipoprotein receptor messenger RNA in hypercholesterolemic, postmenopausal women. *Am J Clin Nutr*. 1998;68: 545–51.

Barnes, S. Evolution of the health benefits of soy isoflavones. *PSEBM*. 1998. 217: 386–392.

Beaglehole, R. International trends in coronary heart disease mortality, morbidity, and risk factors. *Epidemiol Rev*. 1990: 12:1–15.

Clarkson, T. B. et al. The potential of soybean phytoestrogens for postmenopausal hormone replacement therapy. *PSEBM*. 1998. Vol. 217.

Descovich, G. C. et al. Multicentre study of soybean protein diet for outpatient hyper-cholesterolaemic patients. *The Lancet*. 1980; 2: 709–12.

Erdman, J. W. Jr. Control of serum lipids with soy protein. *New England Journal of Medicine*. 333: 313–315 (Aug. 3, 1995).

Harvard Heart Letter, 9, 2, NA, Oct. 1, 1998.

Lichtenstein, A. H. Soy protein, isoflavones, and cardiovascular risk. *J. Nutr*. 128: 1589–1592, 1998.

Lipid Research Clinics Program. The Lipid Research Clinics Coronary Primary Prevention Trial Results II. The relationship of reduction in incidence of coronary heart disease to cholesterol lowering. *JAMA*. 1984; 251: 365–74.

Nestel, P. J. et al. Soy isoflavones improve systemic arterial compliance but not plasma lipids in menopausal and perimenopausal women. *Arteriosclerosis, Thrombosis, and Vascular Biology*. 1997;17: 3392–3398.

Potter, S. M. Overview of proposed mechanisms for the hypocholesterolemic effect of soy. *J. Nutr*. 1995; 125: Suppl: 606S–11S.

Potter, S. M. Soy protein and cardiovascular disease: the impact of bioactive components in soy. *Nutrition Reviews*. 1998; 56: 8, 231–5.

Sirtori, C. R. et al. Soybean protein diet in the treatment of Type–II hyperlipoproteinemia. *The Lancet*. 1977. 1: 275–7.

Tham, D. M. Clinical Review 97: Potential Health Benefits of Dietary Phytoestrogens: A review of the clinical, epidemiological and mechanistic evidence. *J. Clin. Endocrinol Metab*. 83: 2223–2235, 1998.

Williams, K., Interactive effects of soy protein and estradiol on arterial pathobiology, from online coverage of the 70th annual scientific sessions of the AHA, Nov. 9–12, 1997.

Wong, W. W. et al. Cholesterol-lowering effect of soy protein in normocholesterolemic and hypercholesterolemic men. *Am J Clin Nutr*. 1998; 68 (suppl): 1385S–9S.

Yetley, E. A. et al. Diet and heart disease: health claims. *J. Nutr*. 125: 679S–685S, 1995.

Fiber

Behall, K. M. et al. Effect of beta-glucan level in oat fiber extracts on blood lipids in men and women. *J Am Coll of Nutr*. 1997. 16(1) 46–51.

Coats, A. J. S. The potential role of soluble fibre in the treatment of hypercholesterolaemia. *Postgrad Med J* 1998; 74: 391–4.

Fernandez, Maria Luz et al. Fiber called possible first-line treatment for high cholesterol. *Medical Tribune* 40(2): 15 1999. *The Journal of the American College of Nutrition*. 1998;17: 601–608.

Hunninghake, D. B. et al. Long-term treatment of hypercholesterolemia with dietary fiber. *Am J Med.* 1994; 97: 504–8.

Jacobs Jr., D. R. et al. Whole-grain intake may reduce the risk of ischemic heart disease death in post-menopausal women: the Iowa Women's Health Study. *Am J Clin Nutr.* 1998: 68. 248–57.

Jenkins, D. J. A. et al. Dietary fiber, the evolution of the human diet and coronary heart disease. *Nutrition Research.* 1998. 18(4) 633–52.

National Research Council's Diet and Health. 1989: 302.

Ob.Gyn.News. Dec. 1, 1996.

Olson, B. H. et al. Psyllium-enriched cereals lower blood total cholesterol and LDL cholesterol, but not HDL cholesterol, in hypercholesterolemic adults: results of a meta-analysis. *J Nutr.* 1997. 127: 1973–80.

Pietinen, P., Rimm, E., Korhonen, P. et al. Intake of dietary fiber and risk of coronary heart disease in a cohort of Finnish men: the ATBC study. *Circulation* 1996; 94: 2720–7.

Rimm, E. B. et al. Vegetable, fruit, and cereal fibre intake and risk of coronary heart disease among men. *JAMA* 196; 275: 447–51.

Surgeon General Report on Nutrition and Health, 1988.

Trowell, H. C., Burkitt, D. P., eds. *Western Diseases: Their Emergence and Prevention.* London, England, Edward Arnold Publishers Ltd., 1981.

Wolk, A. et al. Long-term intake of dietary fiber and decreased risk of coronary heart disease among women. *JAMA.* June 2, 1999 (281, No. 21): 1998–2004.

Garlic

Adler, A. J., Holub, B. J. Effect of garlic and fish-oil supplementation on serum lipid and lipoprotein concentrations in hypercholesterolemic men. *Am J Clin Nutr.* 1997 Feb., 65: 2, 445–50.

Berthold, H. K., Sudhop, T., von Bergmann, K. Effect of a garlic oil preparation on serum lipoproteins and cholesterol metabolism: a randomized controlled trial. *JAMA,* 1998 Jun, 279: 23, 1900–2.

Bordia, A. et al. Effect of garlic (allium sativum) on blood lipids, blood sugar, fibrinogen, and fibrinolyytic activity in patients with coronary artery disease. *Prostaglandins leukotrienes and essential fatty acids.* Apr. 1998. 58(4). 257–263.

Breithaupt, Grögler, K., Ling, M., Boudoulas, H., Belz, G. G. Protective effect of chronic garlic intake on elastic properties of aorta in the elderly. *Circulation,* 1997 Oct., 96: 8, 2649–55

Editorial. *Nutrition.* Apr. 1997. 13(4): 379–83.

Isaacsohn, J. L., Moser, M., Stein, E.A., Dudley, K., Davey, J. A., Liskov, E., Black, H. R. Garlic powder and plasma lipids and lipoproteins: a multicenter, randomized, placebo-controlled trial. *Arch Intern Med,* 1998 Jun, 158: 11: 1189–94.

Jain, A. K. et al. Can garlic reduce levels of serum lipids? A controlled clinical study. *Am J Med.* 1993; 94: 632–35.

Letters to the editor, *The Lancet.* Jan. 11, 1997. (349): 131–2.

Morcos, N. C. Modulation of lipid profile by fish oil and garlic combination. *J Natl Med Assoc.* 1997 Oct., 89: 10, 673–8.

Neil, H. A. W. et al. Garlic powder in the treatment of moderate hyperlipidaemia: a controlled trial and a meta-analysis. *J. Roy Coll Physicians.* 1996; 30: 329–34.

Orekhov, A. N., Grünwald, J. Effects of garlic on atherosclerosis. *Nutrition,* 1997 Jul, 13: 7–8, 656–63.

Silagy, C. et al. Garlic as a lipid lowering agent—a meta-analysis. *J. Royal Coll Physicians* London 1994; 28: 39.

Silagy, C. et al. A meta-analysis of the effect of garlic on blood pressure. *J. Hyperten.* 1994. 12: 463.

Simons, L. A. et al. On the effect of garlic on lipids and lipoproteins in mild hypercholesterolemia. *Atherosclerosis.* 1995; 113: 219–25.

Steiner, M. et al. A double-blind crossover study in moderately hypercholesterolemic men that compared the effect of aged garlic extract and placebo administration on blood lipids. *Am J Clin Nutr.* 1996; 64: 866–870.

Steiner, M., Lin, R. S. Changes in platelet function and susceptibility of lipoproteins to oxidation associated with administration of aged garlic extract. *J Cardiovasc Pharmacol,* 1998 Jun, 31: 6, 904–8.

Warshafsky et al. Effect of garlic on total serum cholesterol: a meta-analysis. *Ann Intern Med* 1993; 119: 599–605.

Antioxidants

Eichholzer, M. et al. Inverse correlation between essential antioxidants in plasma and subsequent risk to develop cancer, ischemic heart disease and stroke respectively: 12-year follow-up of the Basel study. *EXS.* 1992; 62: 398–410.

Gale, C. R. et al. Vitamin C and risk of death from stroke and coronary heart disease in cohort of elderly people. *BMJ* 1995; 310: 1563–6.

Gaziano, J. M. et al. Dietary beta-carotene and decreased cardiovascular mortality in an elderly cohort. *J. Am Coll Cardio.* 1992; 19 (Suppl A): 377A. (Abst.)

Gey, K. F. et al. Plasma levels of antioxidant vitamins in relation to ischemic heart disease and cancer. *Am J Clin Nutr.* 1987; 45: 1368–1377.

Gey, K. F. et al. Inverse correlation between plasma vitamin E and mortality from ischemic heart disease in cross-cultural epidemiology. *Am J Clin Nutr.* 1991; 53: 326S–334S. 26,42.

Halevy, D. et al. Increased oxidation of LDL in patients with coronary artery disease is independent from dietary vitamins E and C. *Atherosclerosis, Thrombosis, and Vascular Biology.* 1997;17: 1432–1437.

Hallfrisch, J. et al. High plasma vitamin C associated with high plasma HDL and HDL2 cholesterol. *Am J Clin Nutr.* 60: 100–105, 1994.

Heller, F. R. et al. LDL oxidation: therapeutic perspectives. *Atherosclerosis 137 Suppl.* 1998: S25–S31.

Hornig, B. et al. Vitamin C improves endothelial function of conduit arteries in patients with chronic heart failure. *Circulation.* 1998;97: 363–68.

Jacques, P. F. et al. Ascorbic acid and plasma lipids. *Epidemiol* 5, 19–26, 1994.

Kardinaal, A. F. M. et al. Antioxidants in adipose tissue and risk of myocardial infarction: the Euramic study. *The Lancet* 1993; 342: 1379–1384.

Knekt, P. et al. Antioxidant vitamin intake and coronary mortality in a longitudinal population study. *Am J Epidemiol* 1994; 139: 1180–90.

Kushi, L. H. et al. Dietary antioxidant vitamins and death from coronary heart disease in postmenopausal women. *N Engl J Med.* 1996; 334: 1156–62.

Law, M. R. and Morris, J. K. By how much does fruit and vegetable consumption reduce the risk of ischaemic heart disease? *European Journal of Clinical Nutrition* (1998) 52, 549–556.

Lonn, E. M., Yusuf, S. Is there a role for antioxidant vitamins in the prevention of cardiovascular diseases? An update on epidemiological and clinical trials data. *Can J Cardiol* 1997; 13(10): 957–965.

Morris, D. L. et al. Serum carotenoids and coronary heart disease. *JAMA* 1994; 272: 1439–1441.

Mosca, L. et al. Antioxidant nutrient supplementation reduces the susceptibility of low-density lipoprotein to oxidation in patients with coronary artery disease. *J Am Coll Cardiol* 1997;30: 392–9.

Nyyssönen, K. et al. Vitamin C deficiency and risk of myocardial infarction: prospective population study of men from eastern Finland. *BMJ.* Mar. 1997. 314. 634–314.

Omenn, G. S. et al. Effects of a combination of beta carotene and vitamin A on lung cancer and cardiovascular disease. *N Engl J Med* 1996; 334: 1150–5.

Podmore, et al. Vitamin C exhibits pro-oxidant properties. *Nature*, 1998; 392: 559.

Rimm, E. et al. Vitamin E consumption and the risk of coronary heart disease in men. *N Engl J Med.* 1993; 328: 1450–6.

Stampfer et al. Vitamin E consumption and the risk of coronary disease in women. *N. Engl J Med.* 1993; 328: 1444–9.

Van de Vijver, L. P. L. et al. Lipoprotein oxidation, antioxidants, and cardiovascular risk: epidemiologic evidence. *Prostaglandins, leukotrienes, and essential fatty acids.* 1997. 57(4 & 5), 479–84.

Verschuren, W. M. M. et al. Serum total cholesterol and long-term coronary heart disease mortality in different cultures. Twenty-five-year follow-up of the seven countries study. *JAMA* 1995; 274: 131–6.

Coenzyme Q_{10}

Alleva, R. et al. Oxidation of LDL and their subfractions: kinetic aspects and CoQ_{10} content. *Molec Aspects Med.* 1997. Vol. 18 (Suppl): S105–S112.

Baggio, E. et al. Italian multicenter study on the safety and efficacy of CoQ_{10} as adjunctive therapy in heart failure. CoQ_{10} Drug Surveillance Investigators. *Mol Aspects Med* 15 (Suppl.), S287–S294, 1994.

Chan, A. et al. Metabolic changes in patients with mitochondrial myopathies and effects of coenzyme Q_{10} therapy. *Journal of Neurology* 1998. 245(10). 681–5.

Chopra, R. K. et al. Relative bioavailability of coenzyme Q_{10} formulations in human subjects. *Internat. J. Vit Nutr Res* 68 (1998) 109–13.

De Rijke, Y. B. et al. The redox status of coenzyme Q_{10} in total LDL as an indicator of in vivo oxidative modification: studies on subjects with familial combined hyperlipidemia. *Arteriosclerosis, Thrombosis, and Vascular Biology.* 1997;17: 127–133.

Hofman-Bang, C. et al. Coenzyme Q_{10} as an adjunctive in the treatment of chronic congestive heart failure. *J Cardiac Failure.* 1(2). 1995. 101–107.

Ishiyama, T. et al. A clinical study of the effect of coenzyme Q_{10} on congestive heart failure. *Jap Heart J.* 17, 32, 1976.

Langsjoen, P. H. et al. Long-term efficacy and safety of coenzyme Q_{10} therapy for idiopathic cardiomyopathy. *Am J. Cardiol.* 1990; 65: 512–23.

Langsjoen, P. H. et al. Treatment of hypertrophic cardiomyopathy with coenzyme Q_{10}. *Molec Aspects Med.* 1997. Vol. 18 (Suppl) S145–S151.

Morisco, C. et al. Effect of coenzyme Q_{10} therapy in patients with congestive heart failure: a long-term, multicenter randomized study. *Clin Invest.* 71 (Suppl.8), S134–S136, 1993.

Niibori, K. et al. Acute administration of liposomal coenzyme Q_{10} increases myocardial tissue levels and improves tolerance to ischemia reperfusion injury. *J Surgical Res.* 1998. 79, 141–45.

Oda, T. Recovery of the systolic time intervals by coenzyme Q_{10} in patients with a load-induced cardiac dysfunction. *Molec Aspects Med.* 1997. Vol. 18 (Suppl) S153–S158.

Serebruany, V. L. Dietary coenzyme Q_{10} supplementation alters platelet size and inhibits human vitronectin (CD51/CD61) receptor expression. *J Cardiovasc Pharmacol.* 1997. 29: 16–22.

Sinatra, S. T. Coenzyme Q_{10}: A vital therapeutic nutrient for the heart with special application in congestive heart failure. *Connecticut Medicine.* Nov. 1997. 61(11) 707–11.

Sinatra, S. T. Refractory congestive heart failure successfully managed with high dose coenzyme Q_{10} administration. *Molec. Aspects Med.* 1997. Vol. 18 (Suppl.) S299–S305.

Singh, R. B. et al. Randomized, double-blind placebo-controlled trial of coenzyme Q_{10} in patients with acute myocardial infarction. *Cardiovasc Drugs Ther* 1998: 12. 347–53.

Soja, A. M. and Mortensen, S. A. Treatment of congestive heart failure with coenzyme Q_{10} illuminated by meta-analyses of clinical trials. *Molec Aspects Med.* 1997. Vol. 18 (Suppl) S159–S168.

Taggart, D. P. Effects of short-term supplementation with coenzyme Q_{10} on myocardial protection during cardiac operations. *Ann Thorac Surg.* 1996; 61: 829–33.

Weber, C. et al. Intestinal absorption of coenzyme Q_{10} administered in a meal or as capsules to healthy subjects. *Nutr Research* 1997. 17(6). 941–45.

Cholestin

Alberts, A. W. et al. Lovastatin. *Cardiovasc. Drug Rev.* 1989; 7: 88–109.

Endo, A. 1979. *J. Antibiotics.* 32: 852–4.

Felig et al. 1975, *New Engl J. Med.* 293: 1078–84.

Grundy, S. M. *New Engl J. Med.* 1988; 319;24–33.

Li et al. *Bulletin of Chinese Pharmacology Society.* 1995; 12(4).

Shen et al. *National Medical Journal of China.* 1996; 76(2).

Tobert et al, 1982, *J. Clin. Invest.* 69: 913–19.

Wang et al. *Chinese Journal of Experimental Therapeutics for Prepared Chinese Medicine.* 1995; 1(1): 1–5.

Zhu, Y. et al. *Chinese Journal of Pharmacology.* 1995; 30(11): 4–8.

Benecol

Gylling, H. et al. Reduction of serum cholesterol in postmenopausal women with previous myocardial infarction and cholesterol malabsorption induced by dietary sitostanol ester margarine. *Circulation.* 1997;96: 4226–4231.

Miettinen, T. A. et al. Reduction of serum cholesterol with sitostanol-ester margarine in a mildly hypercholesterolemic population. *New England Journal of Medicine.* Nov. 1995. 333(20). 1308–12.

Postgraduate Medicine Special Report: New Developments in the dietary management of high cholesterol. Healthcare Information Programs, McGraw-Hill Healthcare Information Group, Minneapolis. 1998.

Fish Oil

Albert, C. M. et al. Fish consumption and risk of sudden cardiac death. *JAMA.* Jan. 7, 1998. 279(1): 23–28.

Arteriosclerosis, Thrombosis, and Vascular Biology. Feb. 24, 1997. Reuters, Feb. 24. 1997.

Brude, I. R. et al. Peroxidation of LDL from combined-hyperlipidemic male smokers supplied with omega-3 fatty acids and antioxidants. *Arteriosclerosis, Thrombosis, and Vascular Biology.* 1997; 17: 2576–2588.

Connor, S. L. and W. E. Are fish oils beneficial in the prevention and treatment of coronary artery disease? *Am J Clin Nutr.* 1997;66 (suppl): 1020S–31S.

Morcos, N. C. Modulation of lipid profile by fish oil and garlic combination. *J Natl Med Assoc.* Oct. 1997, 89: 10, 673–8.

Simopoulos, A. P. Omega-3 fatty acids in the prevention-management of cardiovascular disease. *Can J Physiol Pharmacol.* 75: 234–39 (1997).

Singh, R. B. et al. Randomized, double-blind, placebo-controlled trial of fish oil and mustard oil in patients with suspected acute myocardial infarction: the Indian experiment of infarct survival—4. *Cardiovasc Drugs Ther* 1997;11: 485–491.

Sudheera, S. D. N. et al. Prevention of cardia arrhythmia by dietary (n-3) polyunsaturated fatty acids and their mechanism of action. *J Nutr.* 127: 383–93, 1997.

Index

Underscored page references indicate boxed text. **Boldface** references indicate illustrations.

A

Adrenaline, arteries affected by, 62–63

Adriamycin cardiac toxicity, role of carnitine in, 95

Aging
of arteries, 63–64
free radicals causing, 64

AIDS, role of carnitine in, 94

Alcohol
abstaining from, 190–91
breast cancer risk from, 182–85
for decreasing clot formation, 76, 174
depressant effects of, 171
excessive, effects of, 170–71, 172–73
folic acid with, 50, 75, 128, 187–88
for increasing high-density lipoproteins, 76, 171–74
interacting with medications, 187

for lowering insulin resistance, 174
for preventing
atherosclerosis, 174
heart disease, 47, 50, 170, 175–78, 180–82, 189–90
second heart attacks, 179–80
stroke, 178–79
profile of, 175
recommended intake of, 85, 185–87, **185**

Alzheimer's disease, vitamin E for, 113

Angina pectoris
causes of, 61–62, 102–3
coronary artery disease, 58
definition of, 59
ischemia as, 59
signs and symptoms of, 59, 60–61

Angiotensin II, for maintaining blood pressure, 150, 155

Antacids, supplements destroyed by, 21

253